Life's Greatest Miracle

text by

Marc Lappé

photographic
illustrations by

Fred Burrell

Longmeadow Press

Photographs in the photographic illustrations are by Fred Burrell, medical and technical images are by and from the following, whose help and generosity are gratefully acknowledged: (Pgs. x & 3) Dr. G. John Garrisi, The Gamete and Embryo Research Laboratory, Cornell University Medical College. (Pg. 13) © David M. Phillips, Visuals Unlimited. (Pgs. 11 & 15) Dr. Lewis Krey, New York University Medical Center. (Pgs. 4 & 5) Dena Marcus. (Pg. 15) © 1992 by Michael W. Davidson Institute of Molecular Biophysics, Florida State University, all rights reserved. (Cell image on page 16, Dr. Lewis Krey, NYU Medical Center.) (Pgs. 19, 21 & 28) The Carnegie Institution Collection at the Human Development Anatomy Center, National Museum of Health and Medicine, Armed Forces Institute of Pathology. (Pgs. 8, 22 & 23) Elizabeth Lockett, Human Development Anatomy Center. (Pg. 16) William Discher and Alan Giese, Human Development and Anatomy Center. (Pgs. 24, 35, 43, 46 & 49) Dr. Edmund S. Crelin, Yale University School of Medicine, New Haven. (Pgs. 38, 40 & 42) Adapted from photographs of fetuses by Dr. Roberts Rugh, originally published in From Conception to Birth, HarperCollins Publishers, with permission of Chanticleer Press, Inc. (Pgs. 32 & 49) Dr. David Peisner, Columbia Presbyterian Medical Center. (Pg. 39) Dr. Rubén A. Quintero, Dept. of Obstetrics and Gynecology, Wayne State University School of Medicine. (Pg. 37) The Royal Collections © 1994 Her Majesty Queen Elizabeth II. (Pg. 44) Carolyn Kaut Watson, R.T., Dept. of Radiology, University of Pennsylvania Medical Center.

COVER DESIGN BY KELVIN P. ODEN
INTERIOR DESIGN BY MEERA KOTHARI

Lappé, Marc.
    Life's greatest miracle: a photomontage celebrating human development from conception to birth / text by Marc Lappé: photographic illustrations by Fred Burrell.
— 1st Longmeadow Press ed.
            p.   cm.
        ISBN: 0-681-45449-0
        1. Embryology, Human — Atlases. I. Burrell, Fred. II. Title.
    QM602.L37   1995
    612.6'4'0222—dc20

PRINTED IN SINGAPORE

First Longmeadow Press Edition

0 9 8 7 6 5 4 3 2 1

COVER DESIGN BY KELVIN P. ODEN
INTERIOR DESIGN BY MEERA KOTHARI

To all my own embryos,
Anthony, Anna, Matthew, Martine and Gina
ML

For Mebbit, Amanda and Sam, and their children.
FB

Acknowledgments

Acknowledgments

With special thanks to E. J. McCarthy for supporting this enterprise from its inception.

— Marc Lappé

I would like to express great appreciation for the talent, effort and interest contributed by Jet Keng to the creation of these illustrations. And gratitude to the following people for providing medical images included in these illustrations: Dr. William Stewart, Yale University School of Medicine, New Haven, CT. Dr. Adrianne Noe and Elizabeth Lockett of the Human Development Anatomy Center (including the Carnegie Institution Collection) of the Armed Forces Institute at Walter Reed Army Hospital, Washington, D.C. Dr. David Peisner and Pat Monahan of Columbia Presbyterian Hospital, New York City. Carolyn Kaut Watson and Ann Rufo of the University of Pennsylvania Medical Center, Philadelphia. Dr. Lewis Krey and Ann Goldstein of Women's Health Services, New York University Medical Center, New York City. Michael W. Davidson, Institute of Molecular Biophysics, Florida State University, Tallahassee, Florida. G. John Garrisi, Ph.D., of the Gamete and Embryo Research Laboratory at Cornell University Medical College, New York City. Dr. Rubén Quintero, Department of Obstetrics and Gynecology, Wayne State University School of Medicine. Her Majesty Queen Elizabeth II.

— Fred Burrell

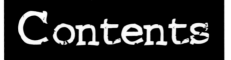# Contents

[Preface]

preface

Observing a nondescript ball of cells becoming a fully formed embryo has fascinated observers since Aristotle watched a hen's egg develop into a baby chick. The process of embryonic development is one of great complexity where forms take shape and ultimate configurations are molded according to unseen forces. During this process, cells move and fuse, commingle and die, transform and disappear as the human embryo appears to recreate its evolutionary origins.

From a primordial fishlike form complete with gills, to one with a tail and paddles for hands and feet, the embryo traverses eons of genetically remembered lives. Ultimately, the embryo assumes its human form, replete with hair, fused eyelids, and an extraordinarily large head, capped with what many primitive peoples believed to be a noble opening — the soft fontanelle between unfused skull plates — which permitted egress of the soul.

Fortunately for those who have wished to observe its transformations firsthand, what was once viewed as an extraordinarily fragile bit of living stuff has proven infinitely more resilient. The early mammalian embryo can be split and dissected yet still retains the capacity for reorganization and development. It is so adaptable that it can survive deep freezing, artificial nutritive solutions, and bright light — all conditions once thought to be harmful.

Today, freshly fertilized eggs can begin life in a petri dish in the full glare of laboratory lights. They can be transplanted to an incubator, go through one or two cell divisions, be frozen solid and then revived to be reimplanted into the uterus of their own or even a new mother. In these new or "surrogate" wombs, such incipient human beings blithely adapt to their new environment and grow to babyhood, unaware that their new "mother" may be their biological grandmother or another woman unrelated to their biological parents.

Life's Greatest
Miracle

It is a further measure of the resilience of embryonic life that immature eggs may be ripened from slices of ovarian tissue—even fetal ovarian tissue—and then fertilized in tissue culture. Such early zygotes can be frozen and stored, to begin life long after their biological parents have died.

Developments such as these are both dramatic and disturbing. They raise major ethical and moral questions about family and the nature of human life and its perpetuation.

Understanding what we see when we look at pictures of the developing human being is a practical, moral, and aesthetic act. Often, interpreting just what the fetus's reactions to its surroundings signify can be an issue of enormous moment. Can we believe our eyes? Is the fetus really as "human" as it looks? As we will see, 10-week-old fetuses respond to stimuli. Some appear to move purposefully away from sources of irritation.

How can we know whether or not these reactions are conscious or merely reflexive? Do these responses denote simple unconditioned reflexes, or does the fetus "perceive" and experience stimuli in some way analogous to the way we would? Can a fetus experience pain or pleasure in a manner comparable to our own? What are we to make of new data which appears to show that a fetus actually "learns" and "remembers" in the womb? If so, is a fetus conscious? Is it self-aware?

To answer these questions requires more insight than science can now provide. The provocative and creative images shown in this book can delight, illuminate but only rarely instruct. The intricacies of human development are now known with unprecedented detail, providing glimpses of the genetic and chemical scaffolding on which the full form of a person is eventually created. This book presents this reality and provides an original look at the process by which an embryo becomes a child. For all that it reveals, science cannot yet answer the question: "When does the fetus become a person?"

For now, let the pictures speak for themselves—with the caveat that what you see is only a partial reality. Eyes appear in the embryo before they can see; hands and feet form before they are connected by bones, sinews and nerves; and reactions to touch and stimuli are at first purely reflexive. The beauty of form seen here presages function. Full humanhood is acquired in steps.

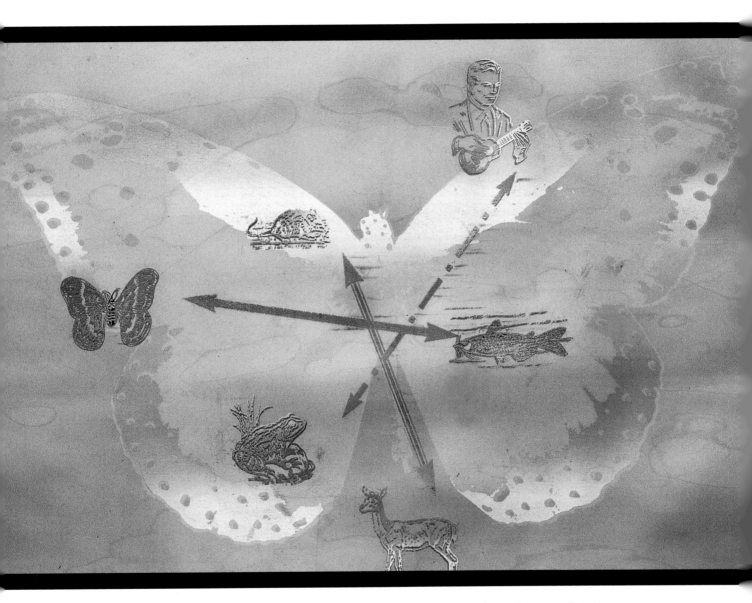

Identical fertilized eggs from different species go on to produce diverse adult forms.

Life's Greatest
Miracle

Miracle

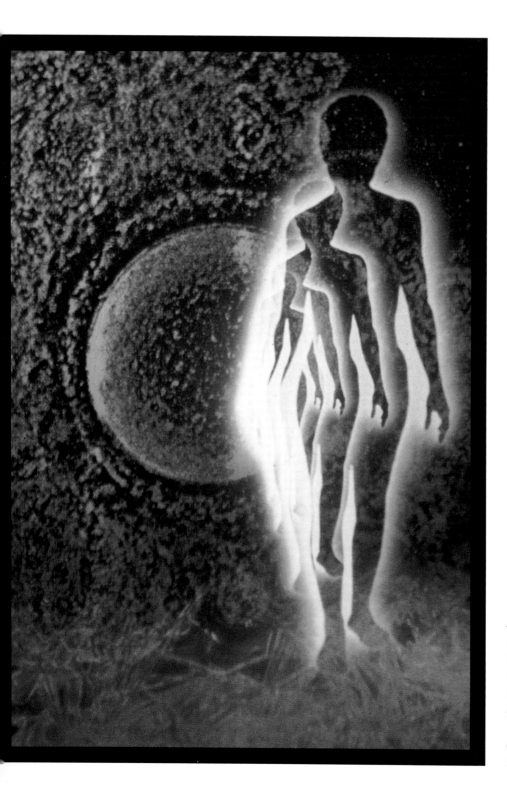

Ex ovum omni. The Latin expresses a universal truth: from the egg comes all other cells. Generation to generation, one mother gives life to another.

An Introduction to a Miracle

An Introduction to a Miracle

The Miracle of Order

In spite of many remarkable advances in understanding the process of development, much remains a mystery. A psalmist once wrote in awe of the miracle by which God knit the bones of the unborn in the darkness of the womb. Scientists have since plumbed that darkness and reduced ignorance and superstition to light. But we still do not know fully how the newly fertilized human egg implants into the wall of the womb, or how it secures its earliest nutrition. We cannot explain why sometimes even the slightest error in a genetic instruction can lead to a catastrophic failure of development or produce a devastating birth defect.

We do not even know exactly how each genetically different fetus escapes recognition and destruction by its mother's immune system, although we have learned to control those rare circumstances — as with Rh disease — when it may not. We know little about the forces that determine when labor starts — except that the aborning baby itself initiates the process. And for all our knowledge, we do not know why some fetuses are born prematurely while others successfully go to term fully developed.

In spite of this ignorance, we have learned how to avoid the most serious catastrophes. Today, Rh disease is preventable. We know how to postpone labor. And we are making dramatic progress in fathoming genetic diseases and preventing premature births. Understanding all of this begins with understanding the origins of human life.

How do we know what we do about the embryo and its mysterious journey toward infancy? New microscopic visualization techniques and the space-age science of nuclear magnetic resonance imaging (MRI) reveal aspects of development outside our earlier vision. Special labeling techniques have allowed manipulation of animal embryos to reveal elegantly organized bands of developing cells that separate one part of the embryo from the next.

Life's Greatest Miracle

Miracle

Learning About the Embryo

From such research, embryologists have discovered that virtually all animals share common developmental pathways. These commonalities reach way back along the phylogenetic tree, making it possible to equate studies of primitive organisms like the fruit fly with those of mice and humans. Intricate studies can now be done whereby individual cells can be dyed with fluorescent inks and followed from their origins to their final location in the adult organism.

Embryologists have learned that in some animals the embryo's three-dimensional organization begins by a simple process of sorting cells into rows, much like the hedgerows of a newly mown field of hay. Initially highly simplified in organization, these bands of cells go on to form the highly structured features of the later fruit fly larva or adult worm. In others, cells organize into groups and clumps, forming microscopic mounds of tissue destined to become hands, feet, and sense organs.

Much new research has permitted scientists to pinpoint what happens to individual cells in the embryo, their ultimate "fate" or developmental pathway. With appropriate labeling, single cells from primitive embryos, like the frog, can be followed from their initial

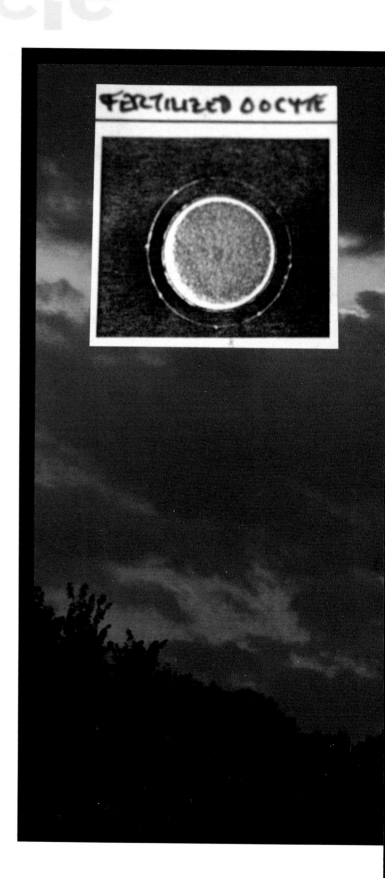

FERTILIZED OOCYTE

Otherwise destined to die, a human egg is given new life by the sperm which fertilizes it.

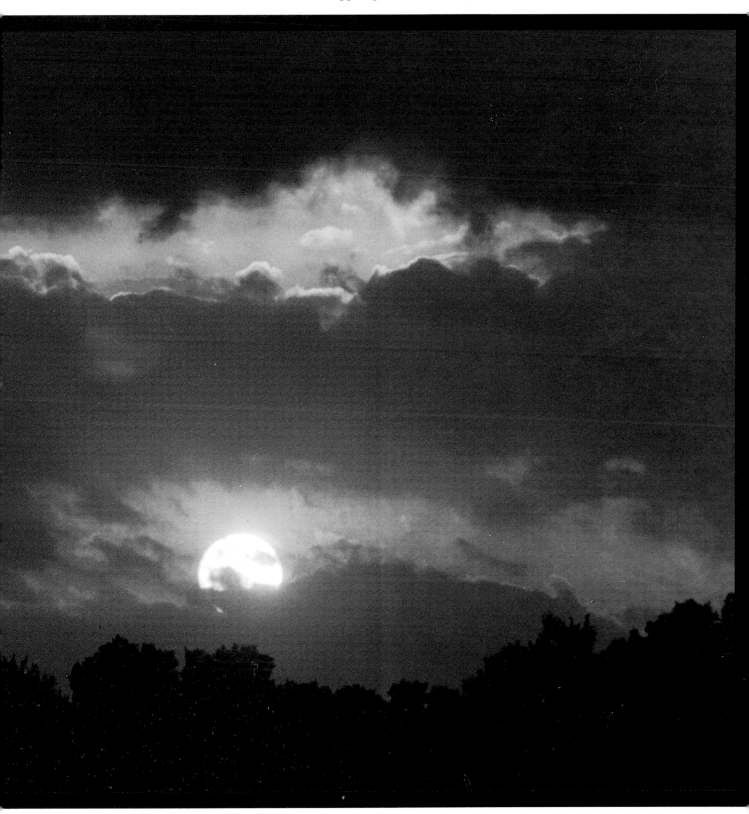

Life's Greatest Miracle

positions in a hollow ball of cells to the final position of their descendants in a complex organ like the brain. From these and many related studies, the origins of the major structures which come to make up the human embryo can be inferred. Of course, this is not to say that a person begins life as a frog or a fly, but rather that the earliest stages of development in such creatures are sufficiently similar to those of human beings to permit meaningful comparisons.

Indeed, remarkable similarities have been observed in the appearance of embryos among widely divergent species for over 200 years. The very first time was when the founder of modern embryology, Karl Ernst von Baer (1792–1876) remarked on the similarities of the general features of early development in all vertebrate species: the embryo of the shark, turtle, frog, mouse, and human are virtually indistinguishable early on, with each one having a "tail," head, eye spot, and somites. The embryos of more closely related animals like the cat, dog, and pig continue to resemble each other all the way up to the fetal period.

We now know that von Baer's observations extend deeper into the phylogenetic tree, embracing even lowly insects which have patterns of early development remarkably similar to those of their vertebrate neighbors. In the fly and the grasshopper, the sections of the somites remain visible in the adult as the demarcation lines that separate

parts of the body. In humans, these body sections fuse, producing most of the skeleton and muscle masses that make up the length of the body.

To understand the basis for these simi-

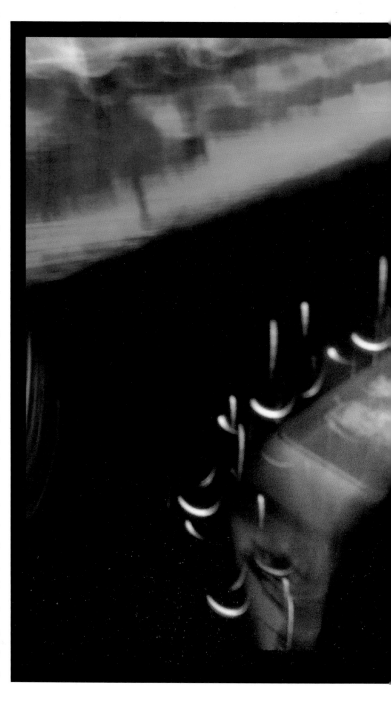

larities requires the simple recognition that each step of embryonic development relies on certain genes, and that most of these genes have remained constant through millions of years of evolution. From the early similarities of form in early embryos across species lines, it seems as if nature has conserved the genes needed for development, often simply by "adding on" as more complex structures in higher life forms were

The genes that control development are activated in sequences that resemble the starting lights of a drag-race.

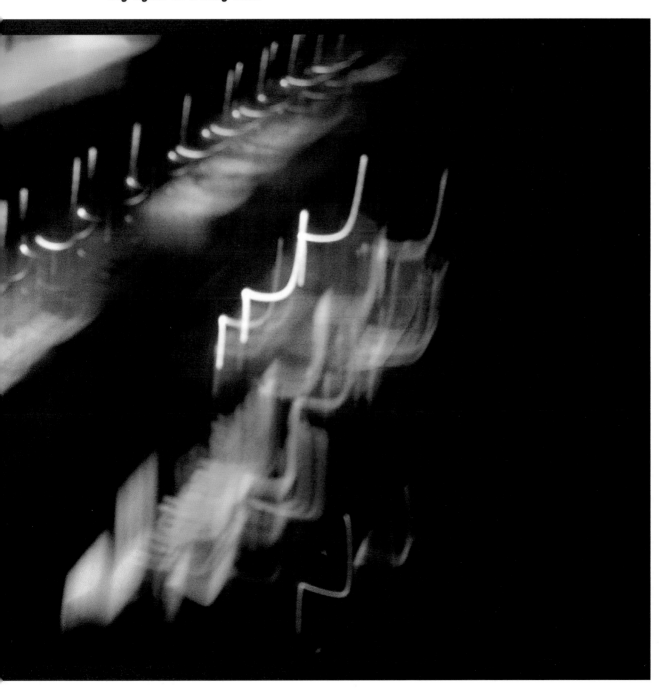

Life's Greatest
Miracle

needed. Perhaps for this reason the old adage "ontogeny recapitulates phylogeny" (that is, embryologic development takes the organism through forms that look like more ancient ancestors) may have some basis in scientific fact. Indeed, the strongest evidence for the common ancestry of all living things is their embryologic commonalities.

Human development requires hundreds of elegantly orchestrated steps. Each step in this cellular odyssey is controlled by the genetic material carried in each of our cells. In fact, the instructions for almost all of the steps entailed in the development of a full human being are carried on four different chromosomes by four special groups of genes. Scientists have learned what these genes for development look like and about the "body plan" on which the developing human is based. The map of development is laid out in the genes in the same general way as is the physical plan of the embryo itself!

How Genes Control Development

The genes that control development are called homeobox genes. These genes are organized in a remarkably simple and elegant way. Genes that control the head part of the embryo are at one end of the chromosomal sequence of developmental genes, while those that control the rear or tail region are at the other. When the embryo begins to form, these genes are activated in serial order a bit like the starting lights in a drag- race. When the top light goes on, cells at the head or anterior end of the embryo begin to use the genetic instructions from the front of one of the four gene clusters. When the next light goes on, the first light goes off and cells further to the rear of the embryo start using their genetic instructions, and so on until all of the genes have been turned on and off. In the end if we were able to visualize all of the remaining active genes in an adult cell as pinpoints of light, we would be struck by the extent of the surrounding darkness: The smattering of genes from among the full complement of 100,000 or so that remain active would appear like stars in the night sky.

This astonishing symmetry between the position of the developmental genes on the chromosomes and the organization of the embryo is one of the greatest scientific discoveries in biology. This new model has provided a unifying guidepost to understanding embryonic development throughout the animal kingdom. Over time, evolution has retained the basic system assuring that the development genes have remained virtually unchanged over millennia. In part, it is this stability of life's plan that explains von Baer's observations that early embryos of diverse species can look so similar at their earliest stages, only to diverge rapidly as the embryo matures.

But it is the genetic constancy from cell to cell that is the biggest mystery of all:

Virtually every cell in the body has the same genes. Just how do cells as diverse as those of the brain and kidney acquire their selective function and "know" how and when to turn off all of the extra genes? Embryologists call this phenomenon differentiation, the process by which cells progressively refine their genetic complement until only a small portion of the genome remains active.

Ironically, the fact that every cell in your body continues to carry these same developmental genes along with its other genetic baggage into adulthood is what makes cloning — the production of a whole new individual from the DNA carried in a single cell — a theoretical possibility. As viewers of "Jurassic Park" now know, this feat may in fact be possible in lower animals. Cloning has been achieved in some genuses of amphibians like Xenopus, the clawed toad. In such lower animals, the genetic material from intestinal cells has successfully been

Cloning placed into a fertilized egg whose own genetic material has been destroyed — and a whole new adult carrying the genetic instructions from the intestinal cell has resulted.

Some new developments in this direction have recently been reported at George Washington University Hospital in Washington, DC. Here researchers demonstrated the feasibility of splitting blastomeres or early human embryos.

Two-, four-, and eight-cell blastomeres were experimentally separated and the surviving "twins" cloned and grown in tissue culture. But no human has yet been cloned, nor is such cloning likely for the foreseeable future both for moral and scientific reasons.

How would we invest the clones of a single person with the respect and the honor befitting a human being? Would our experience with twins be sufficient? A group of identical persons whose existence was contrived by science rather than by nature would be subject to intense scrutiny. Might not the first cloned persons feel like the original Dione quintuplets, whose lives under the constant glare of the press and television cameras proved to be nearly unbearable? To fathom the richness of natural development requires revisiting the life of the embryo itself.

Life's Greatest

Miracle

The contour of a human fetus at 8 weeks depicted by a strip of continuous bands.

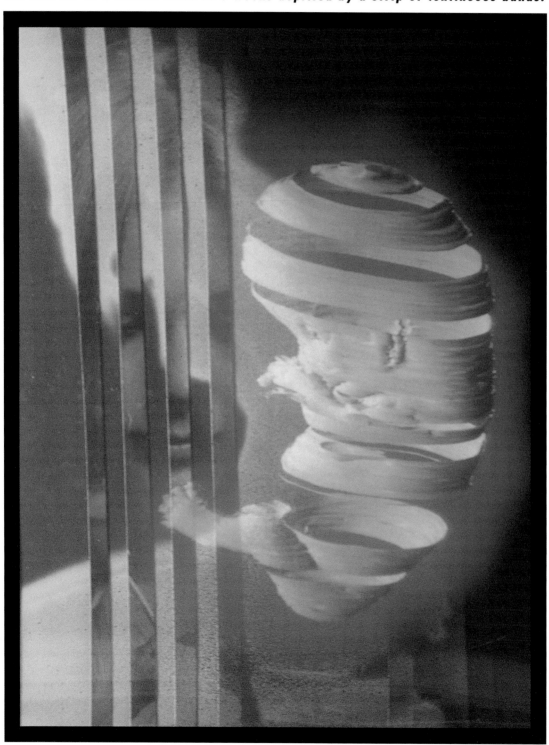

An Introduction to the Embryo

An Introduction to the embryo

Sometimes the elements which make up the process of embryogenesis defy our expectations. Embryonic development is not simply growth and more growth. Even in life there is death. We now know that at times, development is akin to sculpture. As Michelangelo sculpted David from a single block of white marble by removing stone to reveal the underlying form in the rock, so must cells sometimes be chipped away from the developing embryo. Cells die in the webs hiding fingers and toes in early paddlelike hands and feet; they yield and die along the edges of the fused eyelids; and they pass away along some of the neuronal connections in the brain itself to make way for other cells better able to function as these organs take their final form. Without programmed cell death (apoptosis) embryonic development would be chaotic.

Also counterintuitively, embryogenesis is a process of diminishing expectations. As development proceeds, what begins in a fertilized egg as a single cell with a world of possibilities, becomes progressively more limited in its future. While the first 8 or 16 cells of the mammalian embryo maintain the ability to reproduce all of the cell forms of a complete and separate embryo — and even go on to produce a whole being on their own — with each successive cell division, the number of cell types that can be produced from any given cell becomes more and more restricted.

This loss of totipotentiality in a cell occurs sequentially and progressively during development as differentiation proceeds. Eventually, the cell expresses only a certain few gene products — say, the keratin from a hair follicle cell that is destined to form strands of hair, or the insulin from the beta cells in the pancreas. But to see what happens to the whole embryo requires going all the way back to the beginning, where development starts: at the fertilization of the egg.

Life's Greatest
Miracle

The First Three Months

The First Three Months

Fertilization

The sperm traverse the cervix and begin their ascent through the uterus and its connecting ducts to the suspended ovary almost immediately after insemination. Through a microscope their movements appear random and haphazard. In reality, their swimming is remarkably purposeful and ordered. As they move upward toward the frenulated tunnels of the paired fallopian tubes, they are drawn to their target with uncanny accuracy.

For its part, an ovum expelled explosively from its ovarian follicle will be scooped up by the rapidly beating cilia in the fingers or fimbria of the uterine tube or oviduct. From there it will be swept downward into the uterus itself. As the ovum is carried by the fine hairs or cilia of the oviduct toward the neck of the uterus, it releases chemical messengers which draw sperm toward it as precisely as does the pheromone released by a mating moth.

With each beat of their nine-tubed tails, literally millions of sperm race up the uterine tube toward their common objective. Their progress is aided by a kind of reverse peristalsis by which the uterine tube contracts and relaxes, coaxing the sperm upward toward the egg. As it approaches its ultimate fate, the still unimpregnated egg is surrounded by a cloud of cells within a kind of halo or crown called the corona. These cells serve to protect and nourish the egg while it is in transit.

Once in proximity to the egg, the nearest sperm readily penetrate this crown and the clear covering of the egg itself known as the zona pellucida.

As they divided, the cells become channelized into the different parts of the body.

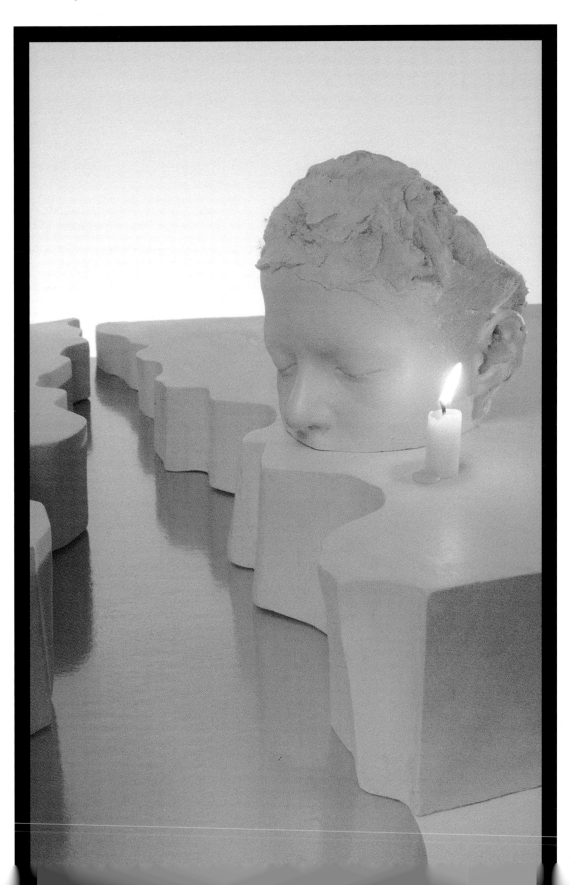

Life's Greatest
Miracle

Miracle

Miraculously, with rare exception, only one sperm head penetrates the outer layer of the egg. Upon the first contact of the specialized tip of the sperm's head (the acrosome) with this layer, a convulsion of chemicals signals the egg to release a wave of calcium ions which sweep around the circumference of the newly impregnated cell. Within a few thousandths of a second, the previously receptive surface of the egg crystalizes into an impenetrable coating. This wave of stiffening of the ovum's surface occurs with such swiftness that the heads of other sperm that may have just begun their penetration are literally snapped off.

The remaining losers in this genetic lottery lash their tails futilely and die. Once inside the ovum, the sperm sheds its protective, shieldlike coat, its tail dissolves in the egg's cytoplasm, and its nucleus fuses with that of the egg. In this way, the raw genetic material from each parent — each with half of the essential DNA needed to make a human cell — forms to make a whole genetic complement and commence the process of embryonic development.

In Vitro Fertilization

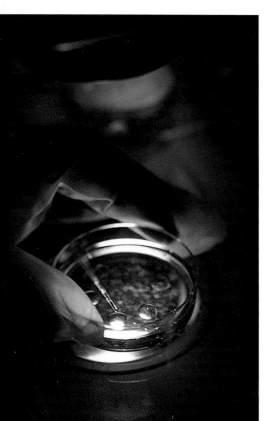

Normal fertilization is not always possible. Sometimes the oviducts are blocked by adhesions or scars from previous infection, or the male's sperm are insufficiently concentrated to achieve natural fertilization. With advanced surgical techniques that include laparoscopy, a process by which a thin tube containing an optical cable and surgical instruments is inserted into the abdomen through a small incision, a surgeon can tease out eggs from their ripening follicles in the ovary or flush them from the oviduct after stimulating multiple ovulations with hormones. Thereafter, the surgeon can mix them in a petri dish with sperm from the father that have been collected and concentrated by putting them in a centrifuge. By providing just the right mix of nutrients and activating chemicals in this glass dish (hence, in vitro fertilization), reproductive specialists can encourage fertilization by mimicking the conditions that normally arise in the fal-

In vitro (literally "in glass") fertilization occurs when donor sperm are mixed in a medium which approximates the fallopian fluid with suitably ripened eggs.

The egg at the moment of ripening, ready to be released from its follicle in the ovary (magnified approximately 200 times).

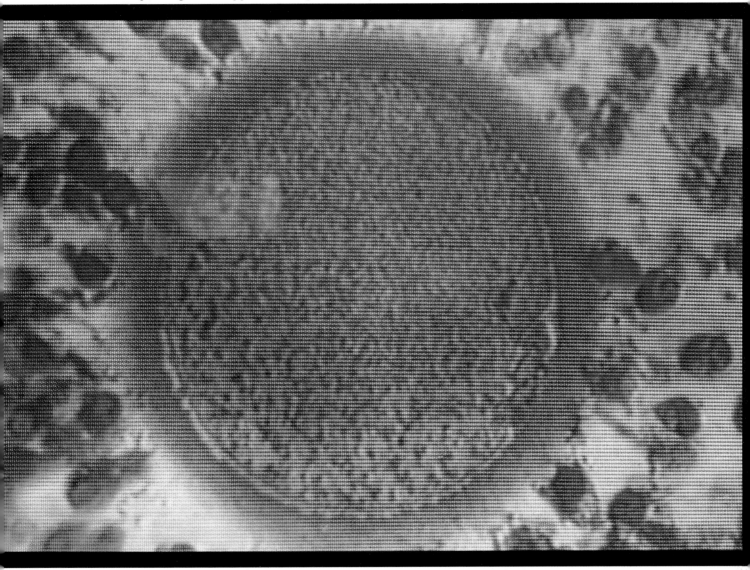

lopian tube that carries the egg to the womb. The resulting pre-embryo can then be implanted into a womb prepared by treating the mother with suitable hormones. If conditions are right, the embryo will develop into a healthy baby with no greater risk of birth defect or abnormality than that experienced by an embryo conceived naturally.

The First Two Weeks After fertilization the two pronuclei of the sperm and egg fuse to make a composite whole with 46 chromosomes. Thereafter, the first three cell divisions occur routinely, taking the fertilized egg from two, to four, to eight cells. During this period, the cells of the embryo become smaller with each

Life's Greatest Miracle

Miracle

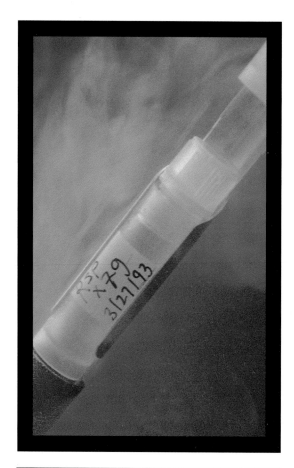

Just after it is removed from a thermos of liquid nitrogen, vapor rises from a test tube containing frozen human embryos.

division, but are still capable of producing a full embryo of their own. If the embryo splits during this period, identical twins will develop. A split that breaks the embryo into four cells will produce the rarity known as quadruplets. Triplets are usually the result of a second split in the cell mass of one of two twin embryos (either identical or fraternal). Fraternal twins come from two embryos in which life began as two separate fertilized eggs. Today, errors in the genetic makeup of a pre-embryo flushed from the uterus can be identified by using genetic technology to test the DNA components of a single cell. Based on this information, a decision can be made whether or not to implant the analyzed embryo. In this way, a pre-implantation embryo which is destined to have cystic fibrosis can be successfully identified and replaced with one with a more normal genetic complement. Ominously, more genetically "desirable" embryos may be someday substituted for those less well endowed.

By the fourth division, the cluster of 16 cells is known as a morula, from the Greek for mulberry, which it closely resembles. Thereafter, a sequence of four or five additional cell divisions will bring the blastomeres of the early embryo to the hollow, ball-like structure known as a blastocyst. By the fourth day of life, the early embryo has shed the zona pellucida, its clear protective outer covering, and traversed the remaining few inches of the length of the fallopian tube to reach the junction of the oviduct and the uterus. In just a few more hours, it enters the portal of the uterus itself. By the end of the fifth day, the embryo is poised to begin the process of implanting into its mother's womb.

In some mammalian species, like the hamster and mouse, if the mother is still nursing at this point, the blastocyst may go into a state of suspended animation for days or weeks, waiting for the right hormonal conditions to signal that it may safely implant into the uterus without disrupting lactation. Delayed implantation is also common in marsupials, and has been suspected, but not documented in nursing human mothers.

On the sixth day the blastocyst rests against the uterine wall, and following a hormonal clue, releases a wave of chemical messengers and enzymes that help to prepare the womb for the arrival of the blastocyst. These substances encourage a rich engorgement of blood and commence the in-migration of new blood vessels to the site. Once attached to the uterine surface, the blastocyst sends a vanguard of fused cells known as the trophoblast deep into the maternal tissues. These cells will become part of the fetal placenta.

During this process, the uterine surface will commonly be eroded, and a small amount of bleeding may occur. The resultant mid-cycle spotting is sometimes called a "bloody show" and signals to the observant mother that she has become pregnant. Miscarriages are very common at this time — from 15 to 20 percent of initial implantations — so that pregnancy is not guaranteed by this sign even where initial implantation has been successful.

For its part, the uterus responds to this invasion of trophoblast with the production of the maternal counterpart to the fetal placenta. The uterus forms a nesting

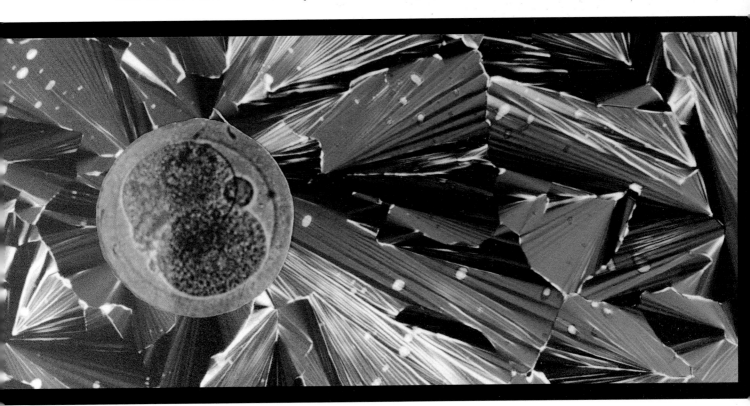

Just 30 hours old, the fertilized egg has replicated all of its essential genes. In the background are crystals of purified DNA, the human genetic material.

Life's Greatest
Miracle

site for the blastocyst by undergoing a "decidual reaction." In this process, special cells of the uterus respond to the invading blastocyst by growing and forming a blood-vessel-rich tissue known as the maternal decidua or placenta. Because the decidual cells (from the Latin for "fallen or discarded") are retained as pregnancy ensues, menstruation ceases for the duration of gestation. The resulting missed period is often the first true indication of pregnancy.

The whole process of implantation or nidation (from the Latin "nidus" or nest) takes place over a two- to three-day period at the end of the first week of life. By the ninth or tenth day, the fetus will have generated a tremendous amount of cellular material in the trophoblast which makes up its placenta. The remaining cells within the six-day-old embryo will have separated into two primitive groups: those lying on top of the embryo known as the ectoderm or outer skin; and those forming an inner cell layer or endoderm. The ectoderm will form skin, skeletal structures and nervous system structures while the endoderm will contribute cells to most of the other major organs.

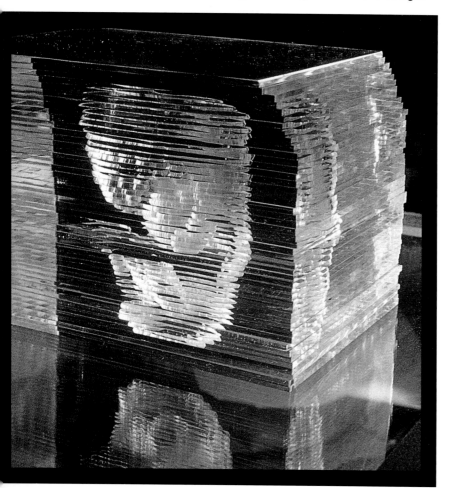

Stacked lucite slabs showing the embryo at 5 weeks of age.

The 14th day marks a departure point where the embryo's existence shifts from one of nutritive self-sufficiency to one of maternal dependence. It is also the point where many nations, including Australia, Canada, Sweden, and the United Kingdom, have ruled (or recommended as in the United States) that any experimentation on the embryo must cease. It is at this stage that the primitive streak along the back of the embryo demarcates the time beyond which many believe individual identity is first established by the appearance of differentiated structures.

The Embryonic Form Emerges

In the second week of human development, the blastocyst completes its implantation and begins to establish contact with the maternal blood circulation. It does this by sending trophoplast deeper into the maternal tissues, forming small lakes of blood that bathe the embryonic tissues and provide oxygen and nutrients. The primitive embryo uses these lakes to dispose of the wastes from its vigorous metabolism — carbon dioxide and chemical byproducts like urea. Within a few more days, the embryo forms its own blood vessels that connect it to the fetal side of the placenta, forming tight loops that interdigitate with the blood vessels of the mother. By the end of the pregnancy, the connection of this hemochorial placenta has become the most intimate of all mammals, leaving only a single fetal membrane one micron (a millionth of a meter) thick separating the fetal and the maternal blood circulation.

Early in the second week, the amniotic cavity, a fluid-filled sac which will nurture the cells at the embryo's surface and accept liquid wastes, begins to form. Later this protective sac will also serve as an aqueous bag that cushions the developing fetus from external stresses. By the end of the second week, the embryo has flattened out and now has a region which will clearly become the front or head end. The earliest cellular precursors of the spinal cord are laid down during this period forming the hair-thin primitive streak along the axis of the stretched out, slightly oval embryo. In size, the two-week-old embryo is just visible, the size of the head of a pin.

The third week of human development is a time of rapid cell migration and is marked by the process of gastrulation (Greek root for stomach). Akin to the shape and structure of the stomach, the blastocyst forms a new cavity and folds in on itself. A group of cells delaminate and form a new layer, called the mesoderm or middle layer. As this layer of cells migrates under the ectoderm, it releases certain key molecules which induce the overlying tissue to start the process of differentiation into neural structures rather than just skin. In the last part of the 19th century, German embryologist Hans Spemann showed that in amphibian embryos like the salamander or frog, if an extra bit of mesoderm — or even dead tissue or paraffin — is implanted under the ectoderm at this time, extra neural structures are induced and a two-headed embryo would result! (Modern science has since described the so-called "inducer" substance with much more precision.)

The head end of the embryo can now be discerned as a darkened arrowlike region at one end of the primitive streak. Cells now sweep beneath the streak in two directions: moving to the side, and down the length of the embryo. These lateral movements also widen the embryo, forming a flattened disk of cells.

At the beginning of the third week of development, the embryo is laid out much like a flat, three-layer pancake, albeit a miniature one no larger than the nail of your pinky. The middle layer is comprised of the mesoderm which will become the muscle and sinew of the developing infant. At the surface, the ectoderm will give rise to the brain and

Life's Greatest
Miracle

Miracle

nerve tissues and parts of the skin itself. At the bottom of the embryonic disk is the endoderm from which most of the body's internal organs will form and grow.

As the third week progresses, the cells of the primitive streak continue to move down the length of the embryonic disk like a dark column of advancing troops. Inside the embryonic mass, the streak sends "marauding" cells into the very center of the growing embryo, forming a tiny tube of cells no thicker than a pencil lead. This structure, called the notochord, will eventually give rise to the vertebrae of the spinal chord. As the streak advances along the top of the embryo, it forms a depression along its dorsal surface called the neural groove. The neural groove expands at its front end where the brain will be, and then elongates toward the rear of the embryo where it will form the spinal chord and primitive tail structure. The embryo now looks like a miniature hand mirror less than a half-inch wide.

In the third week, this neural groove expands laterally, flattening out across the top of the embryonic disk to form the neural plate. Beginning in its middle, this plate of cells rolls up in much the same way you "roll" your tongue. When the edges meet, they fuse, forming the neural tube. Should this process of fusion be stopped at one end or the other so that the edges of the tube fail to close, the spinal canal can be left open, resulting in a serious neural tube defect. At the anterior or head end, an open neural tube may result

in a fatal defect known as anencephaly, where the frontal sections of the skull and brain fail to form. Toward the rear or ventral end of the embryo, a neural tube defect may produce anything from a minor dimpling alongside the spine; spina bifida, an open-bottomed spinal cord; or meningomyelocele where the spinal cord itself is exposed. In spina bifida or meningomyelocele, the child may have varying degrees of paralysis and faces the risk of infections and mental handicap. Open spinal cord defects are also commonly associated with hydrocephalus or water on the brain, where spinal fluid builds up inexorably to place pressure on the brain. With early surgical intervention, a shunt can be inserted which permits the fluid to drain directly into the spinal canal giving the hydrocephalic infant an opportunity for survival and occasionally near-normal development.

Defects of the developing neural tube can now be detected in most pregnancies by a test which measures the amount of a blood serum protein known as alpha-feto-protein. The AFP test is offered to pregnant women throughout the United States between the first and second trimester. Follow-up testing is necessary to confirm the test results and the severity of any underlying defect.

Alongside the neural tube are long lines of cells that run the length of the embryo known as the neural crest cells. These cells migrate from the top of the embryo down its sides, giving rise to the

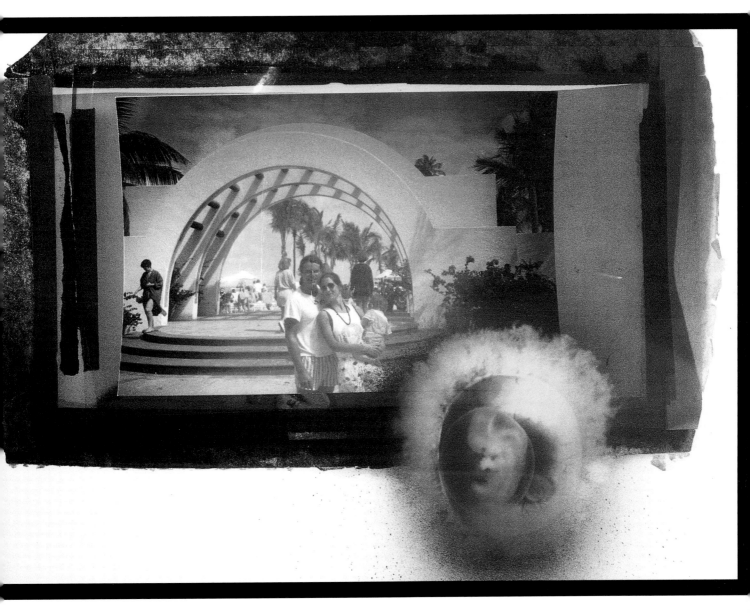

An embryo takes form, soon to take its place in the human family.

lining of the central nervous system, pigment cells, part of the adrenal gland, and the special structures that carry nerve impulses from the spinal cord to the peripheral nerves (dorsal ganglia).

Researchers have learned that all of the pigment cells that provide coloring (and in some animals, the color patterns) are descended from only 17 cells. These cells line up in pairs on either side of the neural crest from the front to back along the length of the embryo. Their existence was inferred by ingenious research conducted by Dr. Beatrice Mintz at the Fox Chase Cancer Institute in Pennsylvania. She did this by putting togeth-

Life's Greatest

Miracle

er two separate mouse embryos: one black, one white. The resulting newborn mice often had 17 stripes around their bodies, much as would a miniature zebra. While all 17 stripes could only be seen in a few such tetraparental mice, their existence offered strong evidence that the colored stripes had come from the 17 cells that originally lined up, head to tail, along the neural crest and then migrated around the head, body, and tail. This model explains the existence of a single shock of white hair on the head of some men and the existence of white-faced Hereford cows: Both result from the death or loss of the first pair of pigment cells.

As the third week starts, the embryo has also become too large and too dense to be fed passively from diffusion of nutrients from the primitive blood vessels that link it to its placental life support. It now must develop a circulatory system of its own which will serve the development of its internal organs. Blood vessels begin to develop from a special group of cells known as the yolk sac which surrounds the embryo, and from the lining of the chorionic sac within it.

The first sign of a primitive heart is now present as a thickening of the central blood vessel beneath the body of the embryo. By the end of the third week, tubes from this primitive heart have extended to connect with the loops of vessels from its life-support system in the placenta. When this still tubular heart begins to beat, it forces blood serum — but no red blood cells yet — through the embryo and its placenta. Nutrients can now be delivered directly from the mother's circulation as well as from the fluid bathing the embryo itself to the developing organs within the embryo.

At 22 to 26 days of life, the muffled pulse of a heart beat, still too faint to be heard by any but the most sensitive instruments, is evidence that the embryo has its first functioning organ system. In some cultures, this moment also signals the first sign of life in the baby-to-be.

Making a Body

The period between the third and fourth week is marked by intense cellular growth and movement. Between days 20 and 30 of development, blocks of tissue form conspicuous bulges along the length of the back of the embryo called somites. These somites — some 43 or 44 in all — can be plainly seen, separated by sausagelike indentations along the length of the embryo.

While there is little visible evidence in the later fetus or newborn of these original somites, they are nonetheless demarcated by nerves which migrate into specific somites during development. Such somite-specific innervation patterns are well known to surgeons who rely on nerve blockage to anesthetize a section of the body. Sometimes the pain from an inflamed nerve root radiates to the whole somite. This often occurs in the painful herpes virus disease known as shingles. There, the pain will often involve a whole somite-size swath of skin some 4 to 8 inches wide extending across the body. The same embryologic reality also permits a simple treatment: Blocking the nerve which innervates the somite-derived skin will also deaden the herpetic pain across the affected body segment. The deadened area represents a vestige of an ancient embryonic somite. Acupuncture points also appear to follow old somite lines, curving along the body and linking organs as diverse as the intestine, gall bladder, and skin along the vestigial lines, following a common primordial developmental pathway.

During the same period when somites become visible, the embryo is forming branchial (from the Greek for "gills") arches and clefts. Aside from a short-lived slit that may actu-

ally correspond to the location of an ancient gill, these structures in the throat region of the 24-day-old embryo go on to form the features of the face, the jaw, the pharynx, and the lung. At the same time, the embryo is developing hollows and spaces inside itself which will house the body organs, the sac around the heart, and the cavity around the lungs. Shortly thereafter, one of the most dramatic and exciting transformations begins: small bumps appropriately called limb buds appear on the side of the embryo marking the site of its future fore and hind limbs. From these amorphous pads of tissue will come the refined fingers of a great pianist or the powerful feet of a world-class runner.

Looking Human   Between the fourth and eighth week of pregnancy, all of the major structures that are the hallmarks of a human being form. The iris of the eye gets its color, and the milk teeth become visible in near-transparent gums. Because of the origins of the major organ systems — eyes, limbs, brain, and internal organs — this part of the first trimester is also a most critical time in development for assuring normalcy. Minor errors or damage done to

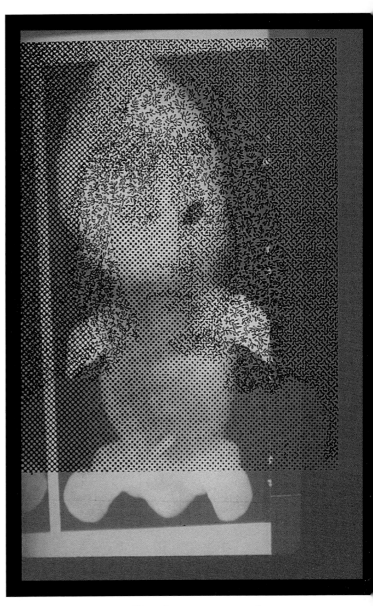

An early embryo's alien form presages its adult appearance.

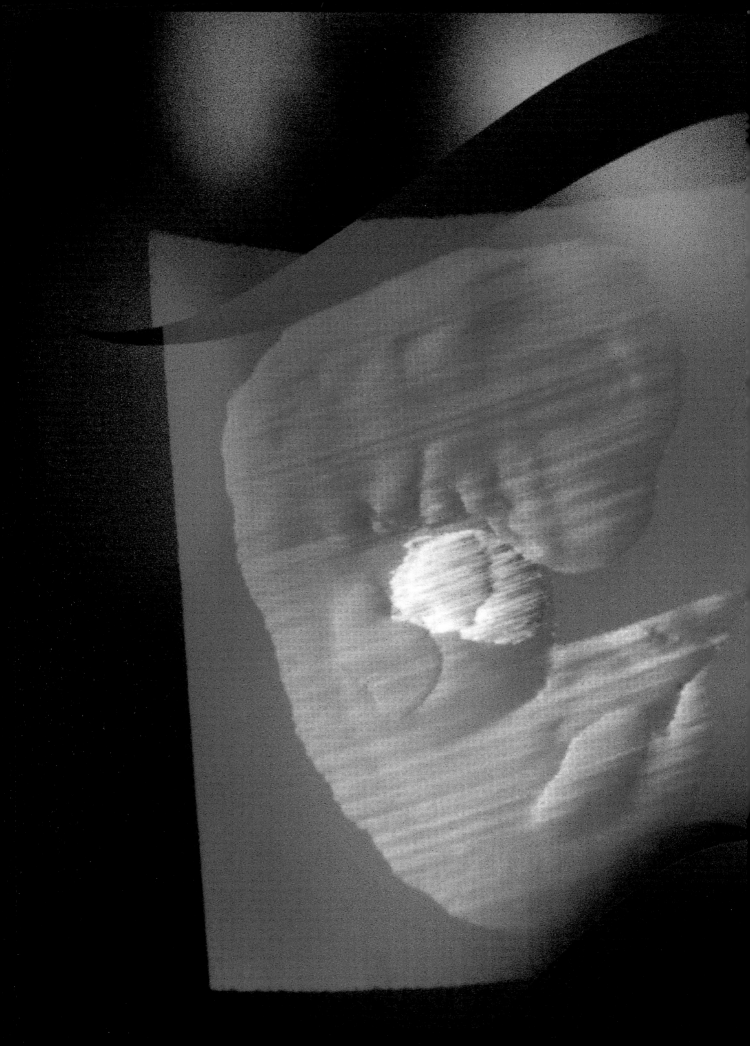

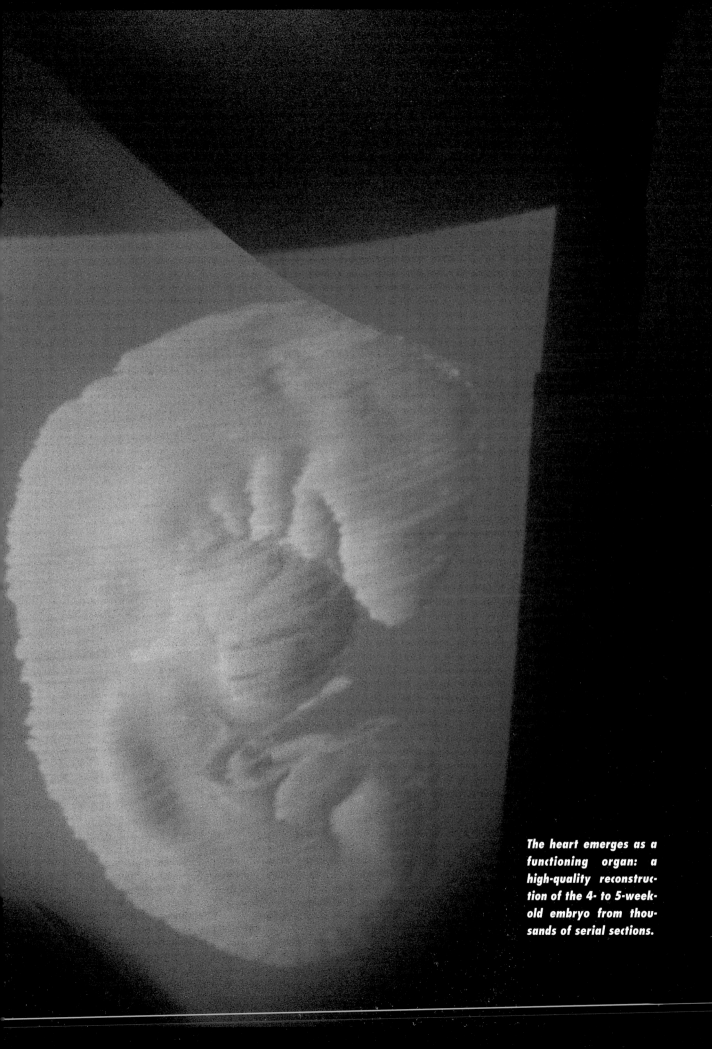

The heart emerges as a functioning organ: a high-quality reconstruction of the 4- to 5-week-old embryo from thousands of serial sections.

Life's Greatest

Miracle

At 7 $\frac{1}{2}$ weeks of gestation, the human embryo looks more like an alien than a member of the human species. An inward shift of the eyes toward the midline of the face, and accompanying changes in the conformation of the nose and lips will render the fetus more humanlike in just 8 week's time.

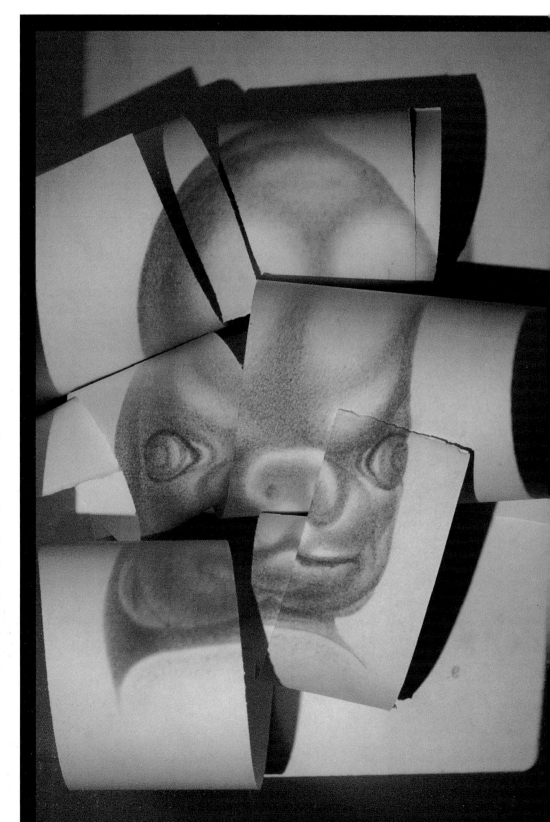

organ systems now can have profound impacts on the future adult. Most, if not all, of the agents that cause organ-specific damage — called teratogens — operate during this time. For this reason, this period is referred to as the "critical period" of embryogenesis.

At the outset of the fourth week, on day 24, the formless embryo looks much like a small slug, lying on top of an egg — its yolk sac. The embryo's external contour is now barely discernible into regions, as wavy grooves along its back separate what will become its head from the rest of its body. But the "head" of the 24- to 26-day-old embryo still lacks eyes, mouth, and brain structures. Just four days later, the rapidly growing embryo will have absorbed most of its yolk sac, expanded its head region, and developed the earliest indentations that will be its eyes and ears. Now along its back, the careful observer can clearly see the string of tissue blocks that will become the vertebrae of the spinal cord.

By the 26th day, the first sign of a limb structure is present — an upper limb bud which bulges from each side of the still minuscule being. The embryo is now no bigger than a grape. By 28 days of age, the embryo shows a bulge on its ventral portion, marking the site where the future lower limbs will be formed. Right now, in this tiny time window between days 26 and 28 is when ingestion of thalidomide, the notorious teratogen, produced its most devastating effects on limb development. Thalidomide damages the rapidly dividing cells of the embryo, striking preferentially at the newly forming buds that will be future arms and legs. It produced the horrible defect known as phocomelia, where arrested development leaves tiny vestigial flippers instead of formed arms or legs. Because the ear is also forming during this period, thalidomide has produced deafness in some children.

During the fifth week, the head begins to grow dramatically. Tiny tissue appendages mark where the future ear will be, and the eye is clearly evident in a still opaque circle of thickened skin. By day 35, the face has started to form, with the ingrowth of the folds of skin which will close the palate and form the filtrum of the upper lip. Here again, a teratogenic insult can disrupt an essential embryonic process, leading to either cleft palate or cleft lip. On day 40, the human embryo will still fit inside a walnut.

By the sixth week, faint rays or ridges are evident in the paddles that have grown from the upper limb bud: these are the future fingers. A few days later, a foot plate has formed, and the ankles are recognizable. The fetus begins to look like a miniature baby! (Albeit, it weighs but 1/30th of an ounce and is barely an inch in length.)

By day 51 the embryo has begun to take on a perceptible human form, with fully formed miniature arms, hands, legs, and feet. A tiny outgrowth of skin marks the ears, and the mouth has begun to form. The face has almost been completed, and the primary palate inside the mouth has formed. On day 52, a close inspection of the embryo reveals a tail! By now, the

Life's Greatest

Miracle

musculature is sufficiently developed and integrated with the nervous system, that a slight irritation — say stroking the upper lip with a hair — will produce a vigorous contraction of the back muscles. The body will twist away from the stimulus.

At about eight weeks of gestation, the human embryo becomes clearly recognizable for the first time as a tiny member of Homo sapiens. This demarcation point, taken at roughly day 60, is the moment when the developing being stops being called an embryo and becomes known as a fetus. The rationale for this decision was once steeped in scientific lore and idiosyncratic judgment. But now, careful quantitation by embryologists has vindicated this decision. By 64 to 72 days of development, the fetus has fully 90 percent of the approximately 4,500 individual anatomical features that comprise a fully formed human adult. The fact that for the first time the 60-day-old human fetus actually looks like a human being in miniature (it is only 2 to 3 inches long!) adds credibility to this scientific judgment.

By the eighth to ninth week, the fetus's internal organs are now functioning, though in a rudimentary fashion. The empty stomach releases digestive juices, the liver starts to make red blood cells, and the kidney filters some wastes. Now, distinctive features that mark the individuality of the developing person become apparent. Commonly, if the eyes of family members are spaced closely, the fetus's will follow suit. Larger (or smaller) than normal ears are also apparent. A unique hand shape or finger size is also discernible.

The whole period from week nine to birth is known as the fetal period. During this time, most of the continued development of the fetus takes place internally. Externally, the fetus grows dramatically. At nine weeks of gestation, the head makes up half of the embryo's body. Inside the head, the bones of the skull are just now forming — spreading out across the brain to fuse together before birth at all but the last fenestration, the soft spot or fontanelle. (In reality, this opening is covered by a tough, resilient membrane.)

The external appearance of the genitals is still remarkably similar from girl to boy fetuses, although internally, the sex of the fetus can be readily distinguished by the formation of early ovaries and testes. These organs are derived from the müellerian and wolffian ducts, respectively, that were originally part of the conduit system from the kidneys to the bladder. The early progenitors of oocytes are already present, prompting some researchers to propose the ethically questionable use of aborted female fetuses as ovum donors for artificial fertilization. Urine is excreted into the amniotic fluid through a primitive opening in the external genitalia, only to be reabsorbed, in part, as the fetus begins random and spontaneous swallowing motions.

The Second Three Months

The Second
Three Months

Sampling and Testing

By the end of the first trimester, the fetus has matured enough to permit its tissues to be sampled and certain tests of its developmental or genetic status to be performed. Through the 10th and 12th weeks of gestation, the fetus's genetic makeup can be sampled through a process known as chorionic villus sampling. In this process, a tiny bit of the fetal placenta just behind the cervix is snipped and withdrawn through the vagina for analysis. Information about the future health of the developing embryo can be given to the parents based on study of its chromosomes and genes. While such testing is usually done with the prospect of prenatal diagnosis and abortion, the hope is that when this diagnostic technique comes to full fruition, otherwise untreatable genetic defects will be corrected with cell or tissue transplants, known as genetic surgery.

But gaining this knowledge is not without peril. If performed before week 10, chorionic villus sampling carries a small risk (less than 1 in 1,000) of producing limb defects in the fetus, such as missing hands or fingers, probably as a result of disrupting the normal blood supply to the rapidly growing limbs. By week 12, when the limbs are fully formed and delicate hands and feet are visibly grasping and kicking in the clear void of the amniotic fluid, this risk disappears.

From the 13th to the 16th week of pregnancy, the skeleton is hardening rapidly, and ossification (bone formation) is occurring throughout the body. By week 16, the

Life's Greatest
Miracle Miracle

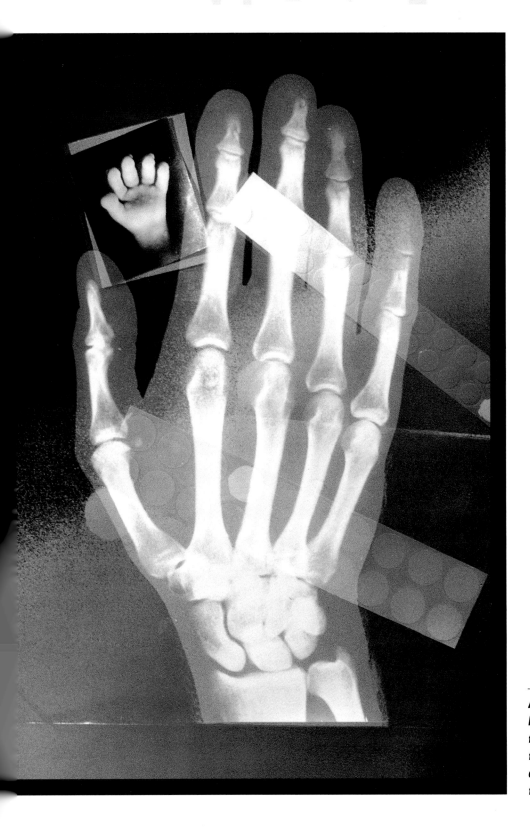

At 13 weeks, the hand of the fetus (inset) has taken on the appearance of that of an adult.

ovaries have fully formed, and tiny eggs or oocytes are already visible. The eyes, which were near the sides of the head just a few days earlier, now migrate toward the midline of the face and take on the front-facing location characteristic of all predators. The 16-week-old fetus has all the features of a baby in miniature. But these appearances are somewhat deceiving, since even with all of modern medicine's skills a prematurely born fetus at this age cannot be sustained outside the womb.

Sensation The second trimester is also marked as a period when motor and sensory nerves migrate along the lines laid out by earlier blood vessels and innervate their distant structures. Fingers and toes get neurones from motor nerves that will help control movement, and later, the sensory nerves which will help them feel. The cranial nerves which innervate the face, ears, tongue, and mouth also reach out from the spinal cord to their targets in the developing facial area. While a nearly completely formed eye has been present since the embryo was about 20 weeks old, it has lacked the capacity for seeing. For this to occur, the cells in the retina which have been growing backward toward the brain must coalesce and form the optic nerve which connects the eye to the brain, and the eyelids which are fused until just before birth must open. Even then, full vision is not guaranteed until some 10 weeks later when the optic nerve is insulated with the protein myelin, and the visual cortex has begun to process images in meaningful patterns.

Movement Sometime after the middle of the second trimester during this period of intense neural activity, something magical happens. Between the 17th and 20th week of pregnancy, the fetus begins to move. This step, known in ages past as quickening, demarcates the passage between a largely passive fetus to one which now makes its presence known. By the 20th week, most expectant mothers feel their developing baby for the first time, turning and kicking, jabbing and flexing inside her. For some, this first movement is felt as a tiny birdlike flutter. For others, it is a Popeye-like jab in the middle of the night.

Whatever form it takes, quickening is a moment not merely of utter astonishment but one of intimate bonding. It may also be a time of lost sleep, as little elbows and knees poke incessantly at the tummy. But for virtually every mother, quickening is a point where the fetus becomes real to her. This moving, twisting being is felt to be clearly alive for the first time. The quickened fetus is endowed with special standing and power in many cultures. For some religions, perceived movement determines the moment when true "life" begins in the fetus.

By the time of quickening, the fetus has grown eyebrows and hair. The fetus may even appear a little plump, as it lays down a special layer of brown fat which will be used as a metabolic reserve to keep it warm after birth. The 20-week-old fetus is cov-

Life's Greatest

Miracle

ered with the vernix caseosa (Latin for a cheeselike covering). This special material has the consistency of cream cheese, includes shed skin cells, and is secreted from glands in its skin. It is believed that this slippery stuff — the bane of many midwives and obstetricians who try to get a tight grasp on the newborn — protects the fetus's sensitive skin from abrasion and any irritation which might occur from contact with the amniotic fluid.

The 24th week marks the end of the second trimester of pregnancy. Now most of the neurones in the fetal brain have formed, and a spurt of brain growth occurs which reflects the multiplication of the special cells that nourish and support brain tissue called the glial cells. It is only now that most embryologists believe conscious perception of pain becomes possible. A second wave of brain growth only begins when the fetus reaches its 30th week, facilitating the development of coordination between motor nerves and their central structures in the cortical region of the brain. Babies born prematurely before this period are notably irritable, clumsy, and awkward until their brain growth catches up.

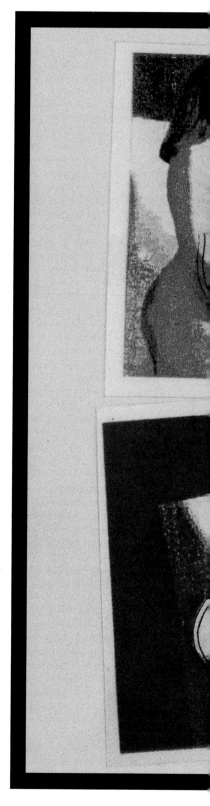

A 15th-century illustration of the imagined movements of the homunculus, or little person inside the womb, superimposed on a picture of a near-term pregnant woman.

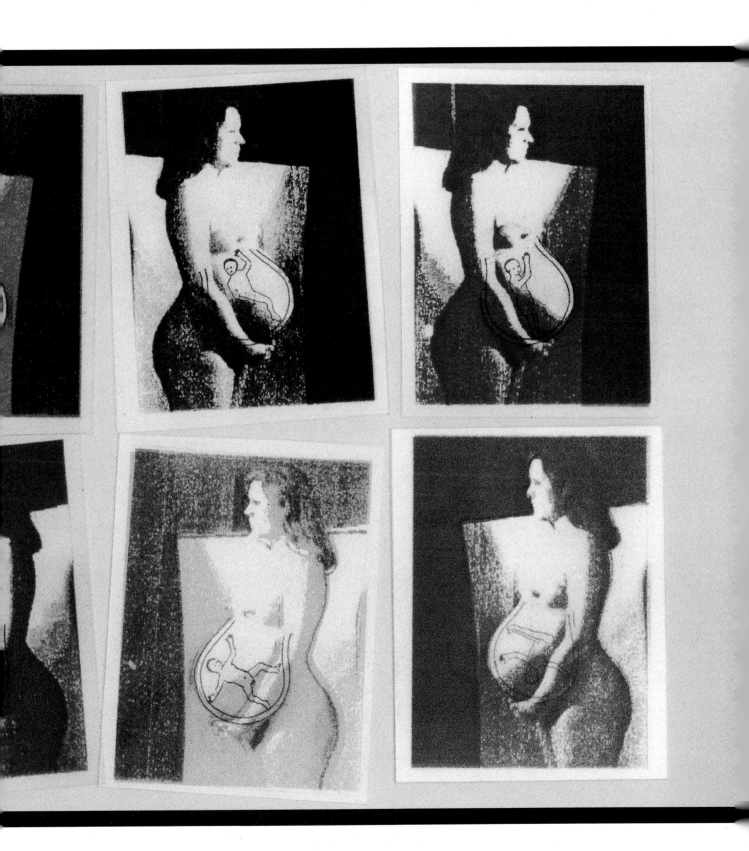

Life's Greatest

Miracle

The foot develops in a sequence of steps that takes it from a tiny, loosely formed tissue to a nearly fully articulated structure halfway through gestation. Sonograms at 18 and 36 weeks are juxtaposed to an adult human footprint.

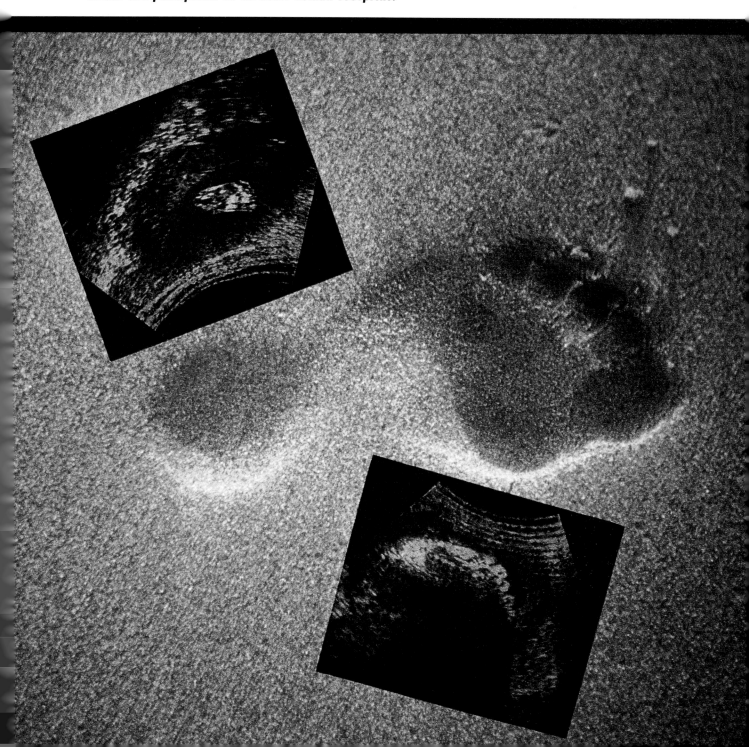

The **Last** Three Months

The Last

Three Months

Achieving Viability

Between the 21st and 25th week, the maturing fetus reaches a critical milestone: it achieves viability. For the first time, the fetus can be said to be a person capable of life on its own. Survival — with often heroic medical support — is now possible outside the womb. During this period, hallmarks of independent existence appear with astonishing alacrity. Beginning about the 21st week, fingernails and muscular coordination appear almost overnight. The fetus gains weight rapidly. The eyes, kidneys, and fetal liver complete most of their development. But even with all of these organs reaching their points of functional maturity, survival for fetuses prematurely born in the early third trimester is not assured.

Weeks 22 through 25 mark the critical juncture between a non-viable and a viable infant. A 22-week-old fetus can rarely if ever survive outside the womb in spite of heroic efforts on the part of the medical profession. Many of its critical organs are still immature — especially the lungs and heart — and the brain and eyes are exquisitely vulnerable to too little or too much oxygen. Even with modern technology, the few 22-week-old fetuses rescued at this time face the prospect of severe physical and mental handicaps. By 23 weeks, a fetus separated from its maternal life-support system, will survive only 15 percent of the time.

Just a week later, the prospect for survival jumps to about 56 percent. And at 25 weeks, a fetus born prematurely has an 80 percent chance for survival. Because many key organ systems — such as the lungs and brain — are still maturing during this period, even those who do survive early delivery face an uphill battle. Only half of the survivors who are born at 23 weeks of gestation make it to childhood without a serious handicap. By contrast, 92 percent of those who survive birth at 25 weeks of gestation face a normal prospect of life. These figures, of course, may vary from hospital to hospital, but they serve as a baseline against which to make critical decisions about labor and delivery — and the allocation of scarce resources in the neonatal intensive care unit.

More than anything else, these data demonstrate just how crucial prolonging pregnancy is during the early weeks of the third trimester. New techniques, such as corticosteroid and lung surfactant treatment, designed to speed intrauterine development, improve these figures slightly. But fetal development at the 23- to 25-week period is still so critical that many perinatologists believe that virtually any means of delaying a premature birth is desirable. This dilemma is particularly stark for those mothers who face the prospect of twins or the multiple births so common after a fertility-assisted pregnancy. Here, the difference of just 10 to 14 days of continued gestation can spell the difference between a premature infant destined to disability or early death, and one that can expect a normal existence.

During this critical period, several tests are possible that can measure maturity by measuring the degree of lung maturation and the presence of surfactant, the special substance which permits the transition from water to air breathing. A non-invasive technique known as ultrasonography can also produce data and images of the developing fetus which can help determine the state of maturity. Sometimes sufficient detail is achieved to permit accurate sex determination and the measurement of the external features of the body to determine if certain hallmarks of maturity have been reached. Major congenital malformations of the heart and especially of the head or spinal cord can also be visualized by use of this technique.

Independence From week 26 to week 29, the fetus grows further toward independence by developing a more efficient red blood cell production capacity and by permitting its lungs to respond to air properly. A rudimentary immune system now becomes operational. The central nervous system is also much more mature during this period, and can control the rhythmic pacing needed for independent breathing and the blood vessel responses needed to minimize heat loss. By week 28, toenails will have formed and the eyes are fully opened. A pupillary eye reflex can be picked up just two weeks later. The fingerpads now have the circlets and whorls which make for a unique fingerprint, the ultimate external demonstration of individuality.

Distinguishing features provide the fetus with an individual identity as early as the 16th week of intrauterine life even though a true fingerprint can only be found near term some 14 weeks later.

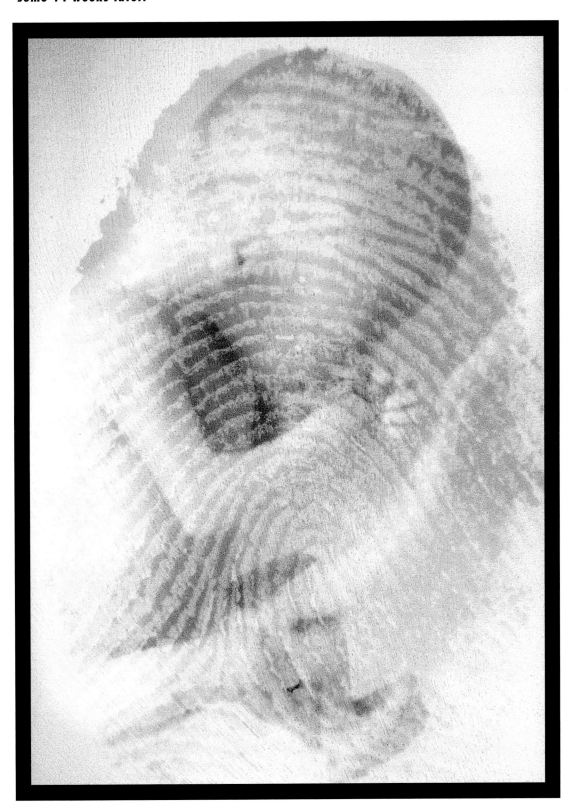

Life's Greatest
Miracle

By week 35, the fetus is usually quite robust and has a strong grasp. It will spontaneously orient towards light if it is not too bright and shun a pinpoint source of bright light from a fiber-optic device.

By the end of the 36th week, most fetuses have gained weight, and have reached sufficient maturity to breathe independently at birth. Two weeks later at 38 weeks, or 266 days after fertilization, barring normal variation or other factors, the fetus will be born. It will actually initiate the hormonal processes that trigger birth by releasing hormones from its own pituitary gland. With a normal, healthy pregnancy and minimal use of alcohol, tobacco, or other drugs, the fetus faces a fine prospect of normal biological existence.

A Home in the Womb

Studies to date show that except for the instance of diabetes, the uterus is the safest place for the fetus to remain. Leonardo da Vinci recognized this when he penned a notation at the bottom of his famous drawing of a fully formed fetus in a uterus:

> This child...is vivified and nourished by the life and food of
> the mother. See how the great vessels of the mother pass into
> the uterus and then into the umbilical cord....

Few may know that Leonardo's reverential drawing actually depicted a fully formed newborn infant in a cow's uterus. Leonardo's professed knowledge of human life might have been more humble, had his views been limited to true observations. Since virtually no one since Aristotle had taken the trouble to look more closely at human development, Leonardo was free to speculate about the circumstances of prenatal life. As it was, he believed erroneously that the heart did not start to beat until birth and that the fetus controls its urge to urinate by pressing a heel against its urethral opening.

Leonardo, in fact, had simply guessed how these things worked. In his day, it was still common to believe that embryonic development was nothing more than the growth of a very, very small person, already fully pre-formed in the gametes, into a larger version of a human infant. So firmly entrenched was this belief that 200 years after Leonardo, the first microscopic anatomists would swear that they could see this little person — the homunculus — in the head of a sperm!

Some 400 years after Leonardo, it was still commonplace to think of the womb as a protected enclave, isolated from the noisome activities of the world around it. In the early 1920s, renowned British physiologist Sir Joseph Barcroft (1872–1947) reported to the Royal Society of England that the fetus lived in untrammelled tranquillity, in a kind of lightless hothouse.

Today, we know that the developing fetus exists in an environment filled with a cacophony of stimuli. Inside the near-term womb, the typical sound level is about 50 decibels, much like that of a busy office. Toward the end of the pregnancy, the blood coursing turbulently through the uterine circulation creates a constant murmur, what the French have called the uterine soufflé, the breath of the womb. And sound from outside readily transfers to the uterus, and may even be amplified by the amniotic sac in which the growing fetus bathes. We know about this because after about the sixth month of pregnancy, a loud noise close to the mother's abdomen provokes a startle reaction in the fetus.

While light and tactile stimuli are diminished, the fetus is not in an entirely dark isolation chamber. The light level is similar to that of a darkened lecture room. Voices and music also penetrate the womb. Apparently, the fetus somehow listens to the daily pulse of life. Even before birth it is being conditioned to the cadences and intonations of its mother's speech. Just after birth, the new baby recognizes the special patterns and rhythms of the language forms unique to its mother's native tongue, and, some say, even

A fetus in the womb? Leonardo da Vinci's classic pen-and-ink drawing actually depicts a newborn baby which he positioned in his mind's eye in the uterus of a cow. Normally, the fetus would be inverted.

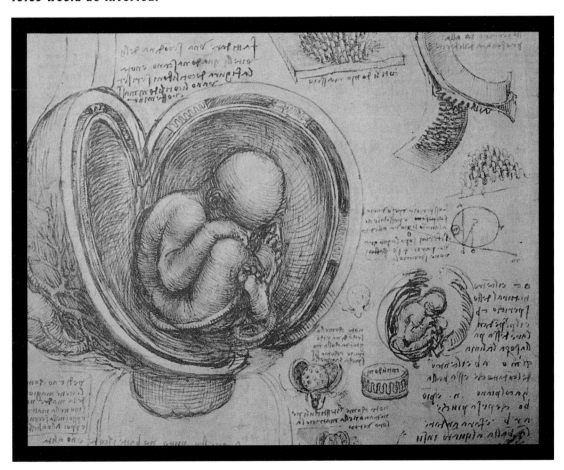

Life's Greatest
Miracle

Miracle

Between 12 and 16 weeks of gestation, the fetus's existence takes place in a sensory environment much like that of a darkened lecture hall.

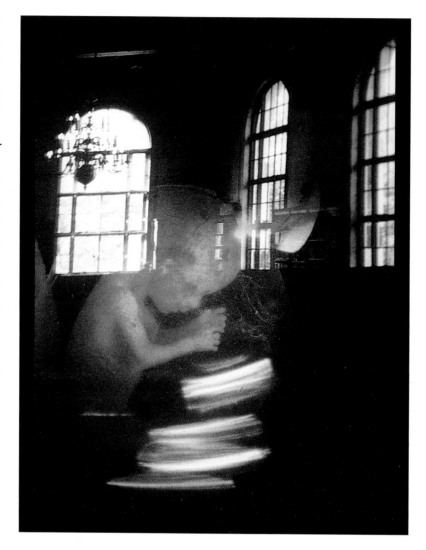

the unique timbre and quality of its own mother's speech. According to many linguists, this intrauterine conditioning, coupled with strong genetic predilections, prepare the newborn baby to hear and develop speech of its own with otherwise inexplicable alacrity. What new mother has not sworn that her month-old baby understands her?

Today, we have the means to fathom the secrets of the womb more directly and intimately. With the advent of fiber-optic technology, surgeons and obstetricians can literally illuminate the womb while using a microscopic viewing port to examine the developing fetus. An obstetrician can peer through a slender glass tube no wider than a pencil lead, and see living structures like the foot or hand, which before were only surgical specimens. Such devices can image the early embryo even as it insinuates itself into its nurturing place deep within the uterine tissues or permit the most refined fetal surgery later in pregnancy.

These therapeutic forays into the womb have also permitted observations of the reaction of fetuses to stimuli other than sound. When light penetrates the womb from the pinpoint spray of light from a fiber-optic device, a fetus will turn its head away from the offending source. A light touch to the skin surface of its face will cause a fetus to

Four fingers of an 11-week-old are visualized through an optical cable, extended directly into the womb. The image was obtained with an endoscope placed through the maternal abdomen and uterus into the amniotic cavity.

F2

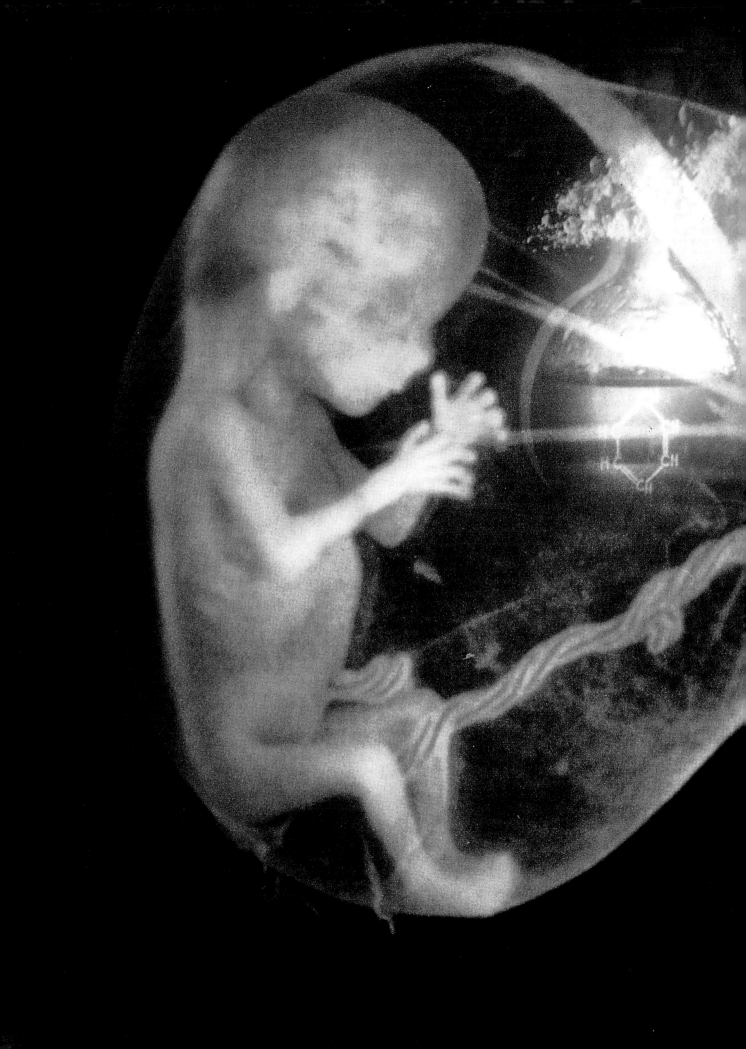

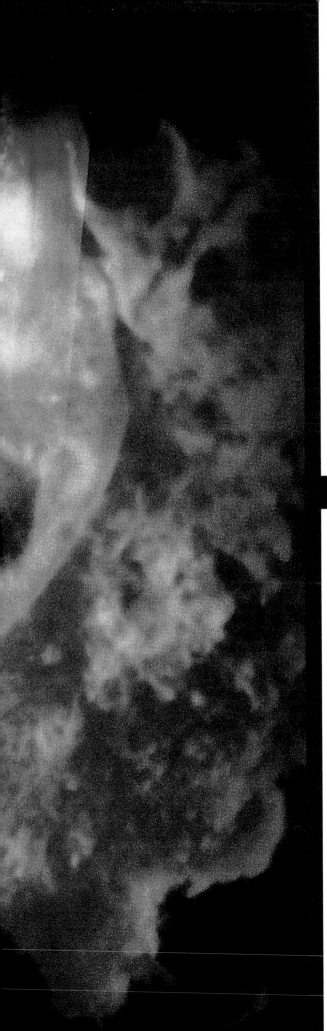

At 11 weeks, the embryo looks comfortably at home in the womb, basking in its surrounding amniotic fluid. Even during this time toxic chemicals can traverse the placenta, potentially causing injury or death. A benzene ring symbolizes the access of poisons to the fetus.

twitch and move away. A fetus will also move abruptly if cold fluid is inadvertently injected into its amniotic sac during the procedure known as amniocentesis. It will swallow vigorously if the amniotic fluid is artificially sweetened.

In fact, late in pregnancy, the fetus may appear to seek stimulation on its own. At eight months of pregnancy, photographs using new non-invasive imaging techniques show pictures of this very little person sucking its thumb.

The Internal Milieu

This image of a tranquil fetus, seemingly absorbed in the pacific embrace of its enveloping amniotic fluid, thus belies a more turbulent world within. Although the first-trimester fetus is cushioned from contact with the physical world, it is exquisitely sensitive to the chemical one. Trace amounts of foreign hormones, chemicals or drugs that would have little or no effect on an adult person, can radically disrupt the normal course of development.

It is not simply of aesthetic interest to see when certain phases of development occur, but of great medical interest to appreciate when and why the fetus is most vulnerable to insult from noxious chemicals or drugs. Not least of the reasons for uncovering these phenomena, is that we now can do something about preventing and curing some of the less serious problems.

With the notable exception of some vitamin supplements like folic acid, pregnancy is a time to avoid exposure to drugs and toxic substances

Life's Greatest

Miracle

across the board. Drugs like diethylstilbestrol (DES) and thalidomide were prescribed to hundreds of thousands of women by doctors during the 1950s and 1960s.

In the case of DES, doctors mistakenly believed that the estrogenlike hormone could help protect pregnancies against miscarriage. DES never proved successful at preventing miscarriages. Instead, it produced a legacy of toxic damage, causing a range of maladies from mild disturbances in sexual development to outright cancer. In some unfortunate women, disturbances in the immune system and reproductive organs persisted into adulthood.

Cigarettes and crack cocaine smoked by the mother can generate noxious chemicals that readily traverse the placenta and interfere with development.

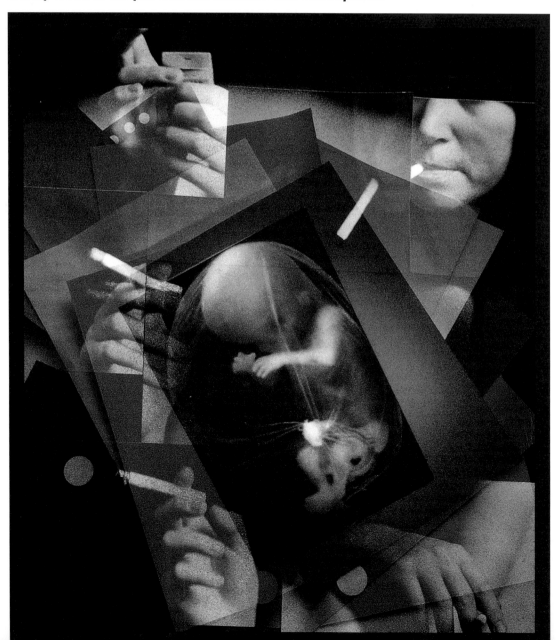

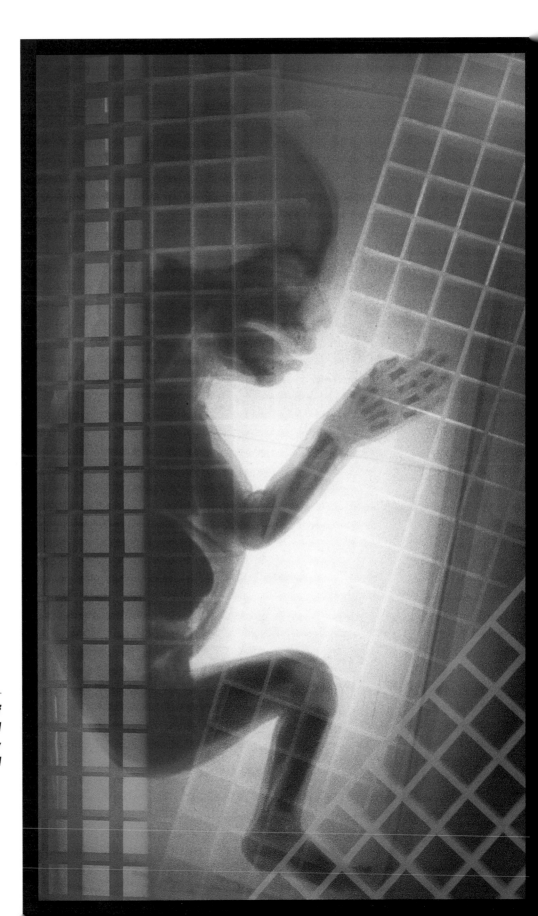

The development of the fetus's skeletal structure is clearly defined in the third trimester.

Life's Greatest
Miracle

Thalidomide, a sedative and anti-nausea agent, is now known to interfere with blood vessel formation. As we saw, it produces its most notorious effects only if taken between days 26 and 40 of pregnancy, precisely the time when limb and ear development — and blood engorgement — is proceeding most rapidly.

Prenatal Medicine

Scientists can now see and measure much of what happens during the remarkably subtle and precise process by which an initially inchoate ball of cells becomes a fully formed infant. Through such visualization, fetal surgery has emerged as a new specialty where previously unimagined procedures such as inserting a catheter into a fetus's bladder or drawing a blood sample from the umbilical vein can be done on a live fetus. In this way, a blocked tube connecting the kidney to its outflow via the ureter can be repaired in the uterus, and early tests can be done to determine if a blood or bone marrow transplant will assist a developing fetus with a hereditary blood disorder.

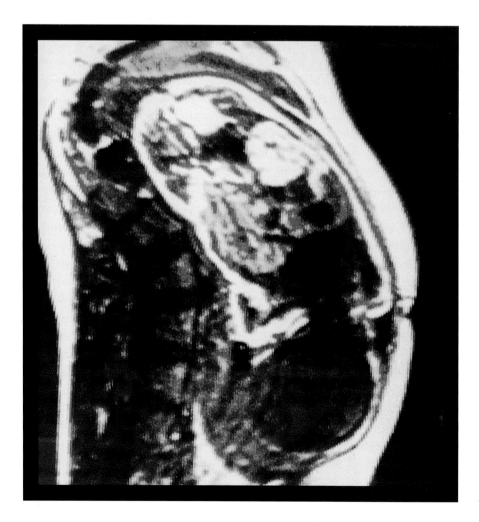

Near term, a rare magnetic resonance image of a fully formed fetus captures the now nearly immobile baby with its head engaged in the pelvis.

Ethics and Development

Ethical questions will nonetheless proliferate as new technologies are perfected which permit ever more refined manipulation of embryos and fetuses. Since 1978, the year Louise Brown, the first successful in vitro fertilized baby, was born, several thousand infertile couples have had their dreams realized by tissue culture technologies. Today, many women are benefiting from the technique of gamete intrafallopian transfer or "GIFT," in which a newly fertilized egg or ripe oocyte is introduced into the fallopian tubes to continue its voyage into the uterus.

Indeed, since 1983, dozens of human fertility clinics have gathered eggs from oocyte donors, fertilized them in vitro, and stored some of the resulting human embryos in special solutions that permit them to be frozen at temperatures below 0 degrees Fahrenheit. The existence of incipient human beings held in such cryopreservation has created entirely novel ethical dilemmas. Suspended embryonic development raises questions of the standing of biological parents who may die; how long such embryos should be stored before being revivified; and whether they may properly be transferred into an adoptive surrogate's womb months or years after their biological parents have donated them.

As we saw, preimplantation testing of early embryos now permits genetic tests for a wide spectrum of defects,

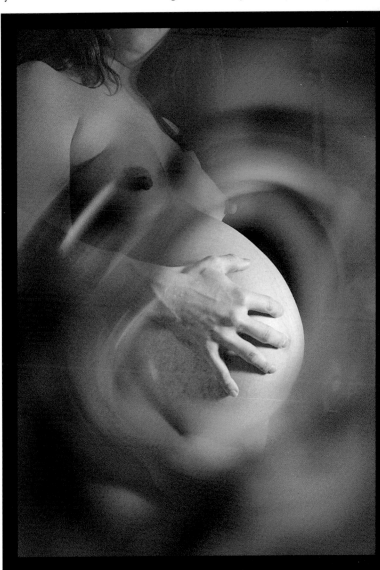

A father's hand feels the vigorous movements of his yet-to-be-born son.

and sex selection wherein "girl" or "boy" embryos are chosen, is already a present reality. Selection based on gender alone is morally questionable in contrast to circumstances where there is a sex-linked and untreatable genetic disorder like Duchennes's muscular dystrophy. Early sex selection, by separating X or Y chromosome-carrying sperm, can reduce the pressure on later sex selection of otherwise normal fetuses.

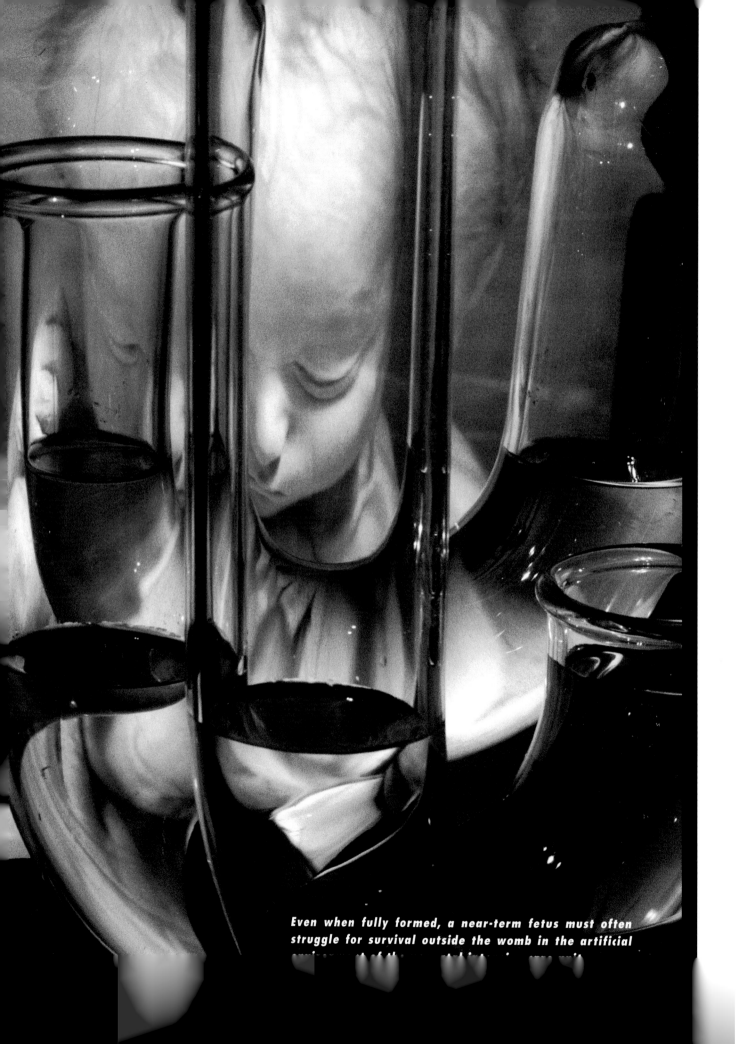

Even when fully formed, a near-term fetus must often struggle for survival outside the womb in the artificial

The future prospect of altering human development clearly captures the public imagination. But are we on the eve of a Brave New World of embryo manipulation? Will some form of eugenics be practiced on embryos slated for implantation into otherwise barren wombs?

Little prospect currently exists for creating "designer" offspring. But science now has acquired new and potentially portentous powers to direct and control development. Researchers have found a special growth factor which will greatly increase the size of a mouse embryo without distorting its form or causing visible abnormalities. Would we be justified in using this hormone to accelerate the growth of an undersized human embryo threatened by premature birth? What about using it to enhance the development of a normal-sized embryo to produce a bigger, more "successful" child?

This slippage from therapy to enhancement has already occurred with a related substance called human growth hormone. Once championed as a treatment for pituitary dwarfism, it is now used to increase the height of "short" normal children. In Europe, technology has been used to permit women well past menopause to carry artificially fertilized embryos. In late 1994, a 62-year-old Italian woman gave birth to such a transplanted embryo. While some countries, notably France, have banned such uses of in vitro fertilization, other countries have not yet acted. When, if ever, is it wrong to be implanted with someone else's fertilized egg when your own womb is barren? As for research, the U.S. National Institutes of Health has recently recommended approval of the intentional creation of embryos for "in vitro" experimentation up to 14 days of development. Recognizing the possible moral dilemmas created by such acts, President Bill Clinton vetoed this recommendation.

What we do know is that the process of getting a fertilized egg to a fully formed little being is a near-miraculous one. Given the extraordinary number of steps which must be orchestrated to assure coordinated development, it is remarkable that the fetus almost always runs the gauntlet of episodic deprivation, toxic exposure, and physical adversity that it encounters in a typical womb. Sometimes "successful" development, in the sense of a normal birth, obscures subtle damage. If the mother has used excessive amounts of certain drugs or alcohol during pregnancy, invisible yet damaging events may have occurred in the brain that may warp behavior and intelligence in years to come.

For all of its resiliency, the fetus requires a wholesome environment for its continued well-being. Obstetricians are learning more about how to maximize this environment to assure such wholesomeness. Most now recommend vitamin supplements with folic acid to reduce the risk of certain birth defects.

When is a Fetus a Person?

The question of the point at which a fetus becomes a person brings the scientist and humanist to the brink of one of the most important moral issues of our day.

To date, neither the U.S. Supreme Court nor any convention of religious or secular

Life's Greatest
Miracle

scholars appears to have the full answer. This limitation has not inhibited those who declare that one or another of the critical stages of human development demarcates the point where humanhood begins. But biology cannot define when a fetus or infant becomes vested as a person. It can only say when such a transition becomes possible.

While science does not have all the answers, it can certainly assist the process of definition. Individuation, in the sense of cellular differentiation, begins at 14 days. Later in embryonic development, some organs have functions which they give up as maturation proceeds. For instance, the liver produces blood early in embryonic life, only to relinquish this task to the bone marrow late in fetal development. The placenta is the key organ of excretion, assimilation and respiration throughout pregnancy, to be totally supplanted by more specialized organ systems after birth. The fetus's hormone-producing system only matures toward the end of pregnancy. At the end of fetal development, the fetus is clearly an entity in its own right influencing its mother's mood and central nervous system activity, increased heart output, kidney function, and the relaxation of the pelvic ligaments.

In contrast to some traditional legalistic views which posit that the fetus is always "part of" its mother, the developmental picture that emerges shows the fetus to be separate from its mother physiologically, yet highly dependent on her self-care and well-being for its continued existence. The fetus is a unique biological entity, an individual by all rights, but an individual that relies entirely on its mother's nurturing through at least the first 22 weeks of life. Until this period of fetal development is completed, say at week 23, it is completely dependent on both its mother and external support systems to attain an independent existence. This is what is meant by "viability."

Perhaps to defer the grief brought about by high infant mortality, some cultures do not consider a child to be a fully vested being until it reaches the age of five years (Inuit, Eskimo); or six years, six months, six weeks, and six days (Japanese, Hawaiian). In other cultures, the fetus is deemed to be a full human being from the moment of conception. Thus, we have no cross-cultural, universal determination of the timing and status of the fetus as a person, or when that person achieves full legal and moral standing. Given this cultural variability, the delicate designation of personhood is an issue that is informed by, but best left outside of, the bounds of science.

The Embryo in Modern Times

By opening a Pandora's box of new possibilities, modern embryologic science has created a plethora of new problems that inevitably will change the conceptualization of personhood. The enormous latitude for manipulation in early development, which we have reviewed in this book, raises concerns over who best controls the first

With its head firmly engaged in the pelvis, the fetus is ready to begin the process of birthing.

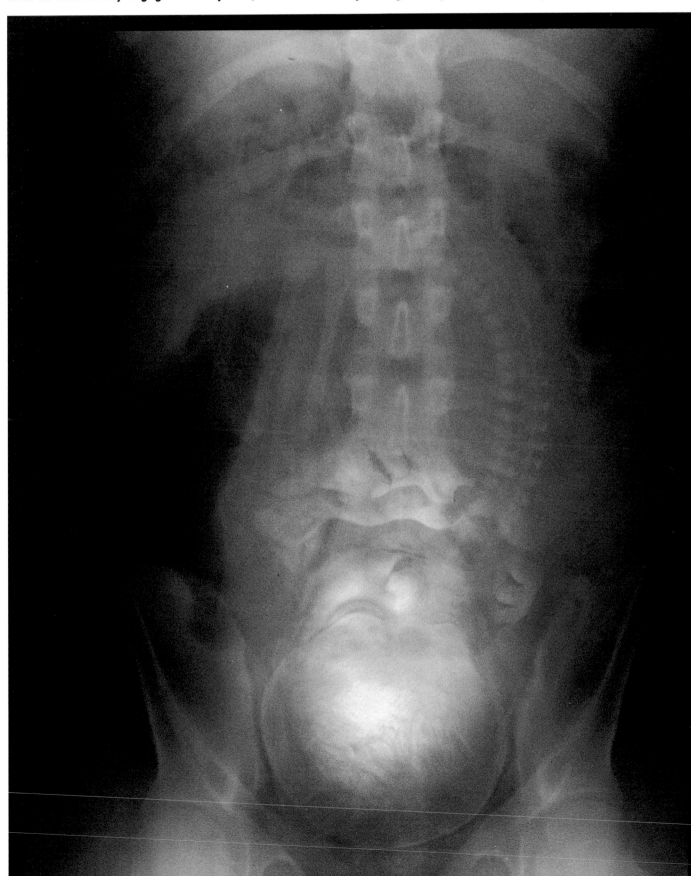

Life's Greatest
Miracle

stages of life. Prenatal geneticists, fetologists, and perinatologists will make up a new cadre of 21st-century medical practitioners. And adoptive parents, surrogate mothers, and new biological partners, unconnected by traditional, biologically based bonds of love and fidelity will become the reality of human medicine in the year 2000. Even then the ultimate success of embryologic development will still be a thing of wonder. For the human infant to be seen as anything other than a miracle — is to ask too much of science and too little of the unspoken hand of forces still beyond our ken. In the end, it may be critical to remember that while a life may begin in the womb, its full fruition comes not at birth, but only years later, after much love, turmoil, and individual choice.

Glossary

Acrosome. The enzyme-packed area in the head of a sperm that helps activate the ovum during fertilization.

Anencephaly. An invariably fatal defect in brain and skull development caused by the failure of the neural tube to close at its anterior end.

Alpha-fetoprotein. A serum protein whose elevation can signal the presence of a neural tube birth defect.

Anterior. Referring to the front or head end; the most forward part.

Apoptosis. A genetically programmed process by which cells initiate their own death.

Blastomeres. The identical cells which arise shortly after fertilization that comprise the 6- to 8-cell pre-embryo.

Blastocyst. The hollow ball of cells that implants into the uterine wall.

Branchial. Referring to the areas in the anterior end of the embryo during the early part of the embryonic period which will give rise to the structures of the face and neck.

Chorionic villus sampling (C.V.S.). The testing process by which small pieces of the fingers of the fetal placenta are sampled through the cervix, usually during weeks 10 to 12 of development.

Cleft palate/lip. A birth defect of the face which results from the incomplete fusion of embryonic plates.

Cloning. A method whereby the genetic information of a single cell is perpetuated through the propagation of the descendants of that cell; in the instance of an early embryo, the process of creating duplicate embryos by encouraging the growth of one or more blastomeres.

Congenital malformation. A birth defect apparent at birth.

Corona. The "crown" or group of cells which surround and nourish the ovum after it is released from its follicle.

Critical period. The stages during the first trimester of pregnancy during which organs are most actively forming.

Decidua. The maternal portion of the placenta; or, the cells which make up that placental tissue (c.f. decidual cells).

Diethylstilbestrol (DES). A potent, estrogenlike, non-steroidal hormone prescribed for women in the 1950s and 1960s in a misguided attempt to prevent miscarriages; the teratogen of the same name.

Differentiation. The process by which simple embryonic cells become more and more specialized in their functions.

Dorsum. Referring to the top of the embryo (c.f. the dorsal area).

Dorsal ganglia. The nerve root centers that extend from the edges of the vertebrae.

Fetal period. The stage of development when the embryo first takes on human features; approximately 60 days after fertilization up to birth.

Gastrulation. The process by which cells in the blastocyst migrate inward to form a cavity and induce the head structures of the embryo to form.

Glial cells. The cells which surround and support the neurones in the brain; also known as neuroglial cells.

Homeobox. The area on the fourth chromosome which includes at least four different gene groups that control the staging of embryonic development.

In vitro fertilization. The procedure of combining sperm and ova in tissue culture.

Laparoscopy. A small surgical incision through which viewing devices or surgical instruments may be inserted to view the internal organs or uterine contents.

Lateral. Referring to the sides of an organ or structure.

Limb bud. A slightly bulging, bilateral area of cells along the edge of the 25- to 30-day embryo which will produce the structures of the arms and legs.

Lung surfactant. A proteinaceous material which assists the lung to accommodate air contact after birth.

Meningomyelocele. An open, cystlike structural defect of the spine.

Mesoderm. The middle cell layer of the early embryo which gives rise to muscle and other body cells.

Morula. The very early (2- to 3-day) embryo which resembles a mulberry or raspberry.

Müellerian ducts. The tubular structures which go alongside the early kidney that gives rise to the ovary, oviduct or uterine tube, the uterus, and the vagina.

Myelin. The proteinaceous lining that insulates most nerves.

Neural tube. The structure which runs along the back or dorsum of the early embryo which will give rise to the spinal cord (c.f. neural tube defects).

Neural tube defects. Congenital malformations which arise from the failure of the neural tube to close at one end or the other (c.f. anencephaly and spina bifida).

Nidation. The process of implantation by which the blastocyst lodges in the uterine wall.

Notochord. The primitive structure from which the spinal column will form.

Oocytes. The (usually) immature egg cells that go on to become ova.

Optic. Referring to the eye (e.g., the optic cup which gives rise to the retina).

Otic. Referring to the ear (e.g., the otic vesicle which gives rise to the ear).

Ova. Eggs.

Phocomelia. Incomplete or absent development of the limbs.

Placenta. The organ which nourishes the embryo and fetus.

Pre-embryo. The earliest stages of development after fertilization before the appearance of any discernible structures; the first 14 days of embryonic development.

Quickening. The date when movement of the fetus is first perceived by the mother, usually around the 17th week of pregnancy.

Rh disease. Also known as erythroblastosis fetalis. A red-blood cell destroying process caused by the presence of maternal antibodies to fetal red blood cells that express the Rh antigen; preventable by treating Rh negative mothers with Rh gamma globulin at the end of a pregnancy with an Rh positive fetus.

ex selection. The process by which an embryo of a given sex is chosen ough any of several means, including preferential fertilization with X or Y chromosome bearing sperm; destruction of XX or XY pre-embryos; or abortion of an embryo or early fetus of a given sex.

Somite. Any one of 43 distinct surface elevations along the dorsum of the 20- to 30-day embryo which will give rise to the vertebral column, ribs, sternum, and skull; their musculature; and the associated skin and dermal structures.

Teratogen. An agent, usually viral, chemical or metallic, capable of producing a birth defect.

Thalidomide. A potent sedative known to produce human birth defects.

Totipotential. Referring to the capacity of a given cell, usually from a pre-embryo, to produce all of the cell types of the adult.

Trophoblast. The extra-embryonic cells of the early embryo which invade the uterus and produce the cells of the fetal placenta.

Ultrasonography. A noninvasive procedure by which high-frequency sound waves are used to visualize the fetus.

Vernix caseosa. The slick covering that helps protect the term fetus during delivery.

Visual cortex. The area of the brain associated with vision.

Yolk sac. A vestigial structure which surrounds the early embryo and contributes blood cells and vessels to the developing blood supply system.

Zona pellucida. The clear, tough covering that surrounds the early blastocyst.

Zygote. The fertilized egg.